Mummy doesn't love you

Mummy doesn't love you

The shocking true story of a mother's campaign to destroy the mind and life of her own child

Alexander Sinclair

EBURY
PRESS

Alexander Sinclair is a pseudonym.

5 7 9 10 8 6 4

Published in 2009 by Ebury Press, an imprint of Ebury Publishing
A Random House Group company

Copyright © Alexander Sinclair 2009

Alexander Sinclair has asserted his right to be identified as
the author of this Work in accordance with the Copyright,
Designs and Patents Act 1988

The Random House Group Limited Reg. No. 954009

Addresses for companies within the Random House Group can be
found at www.randomhouse.co.uk

A CIP catalogue record for this book is available from
the British Library

The Random House Group Limited supports The Forest Stewardship
Council (FSC), the leading international forest certification
organisation. All our titles that are printed on Greenpeace approved
FSC certified paper carry the FSC logo. Our paper procurement
policy can be found at www.rbooks.co.uk/environment

Printed in the UK by CPI Cox & Wyman, Reading, RG1 8EX

ISBN 9780091928070

To buy books by your favourite authors and register for offers visit
www.rbooks.co.uk

*To my father, whose forbearance and perseverance
undoubtedly saved my life*

Disclaimer

This book is a work of non-fiction based on the life, experiences and recollections of the author. In some limited cases names of people, places, dates, sequences or the detail of events have been changed to protect the privacy of others.

Contents

Prologue

Hard hands grasped my shoulders and propelled me down the dark corridor. Before me were six doors to six isolation cells. I cried out to the man not to throw me in, but he took no notice, just gave me a hard shake and kneed me in the back as he forced me along. Another man ran ahead, opened one of the heavy pale-blue doors, and it gaped before me, heralding, I knew, the horrors to come: isolation by myself and a long, pitch-dark night.

I refused to go in and tried to hold myself back, my bare feet slipping on the floor, just to receive another knee in the small of my back and a hard cuff across my head to make me move. I sobbed and let my legs collapse under me and flopped on the ground. The two men grasped my arms and dragged me into the room, where I was dumped on the floor. They retreated, slamming the door behind them.

I lifted my head, and beheld the pale small form of a child lying in the middle of the room; I knew who it was, I knew what was to come. I let out a scream, and jerked awake ...

I had had my nightmare again, the nightmare that has plagued me for nearly thirty-five years, ever since I was ten years old.

When the nights, darkness, and sleep, can take you back to the worst possible nightmare, there is nowhere safe, no one who can help you. Even your waking hours can be terrifying, where the slightest event can precipitate the most dreadful flashbacks, and you become isolated in a crowded room, a prisoner of your own mind.

After my father rescued me from the institution, I was afraid to be with people; I was afraid to be alone; I was afraid to be in a crowd; I was afraid of the dark. I was even afraid of falling asleep. The only place I felt safe was with my father, but he could not be there for me twenty-four hours a day.

Throughout the remainder of my childhood, I slept with the light on. In the days following my rescue I was too mentally damaged to understand – too damaged to control – the debilitating mental trauma that was a result of my time in the institution. I used to lie in my bed every night taking turns to hold an arm straight above my head, reasoning that if I fell asleep my arm would drop on my head and wake me again. It never really worked; I eventually fell asleep to suffer my nightmare once again. Even now, many years later, the nightmares will sneak up and haunt me when I least expect it, breaking into the happy and stable life I have built for myself. And the person responsible for all this trauma, damage, and terror, was my own mother.

How did I end up locked away in an institution at the tender age of ten? Why did my mother want to separate me from my family and to brand me as severely mentally impaired and emotionally unstable? Why did she hate me so much that my life became one of anguish and despair? It didn't help me that my mother had manipulated and tricked my father and that he believed her lies. In our society women are meant to be nurturers, to uphold family values, but my mother hated me with unrelenting fervour, and ultimately it became all the easier for her to use me as a pawn in the power play against my father.

If it had not been for my mother's campaign of psychological warfare against me, I would have been a normal child, with strengths and weaknesses like anybody else. However, I lived my childhood in a state of constant fear of my mother, and this made me insecure and fearful. When I had problems at school, I was mistakenly labelled backward. Day after day I was told I was mental, autistic, retarded and was destined to end up in more than one mental institution. Yet after my mother's control – her abuse – of me ended, my true personality began to emerge. I turned out a sensitive and kind person. I took a degree at university, and ultimately became a professional author and married in a loving relationship.

After what I went through as a child it has always been difficult for me to look back on my early life and see myself for what I was: a normal child who was terrorised by the person who is supposed to love and nurture you. I've since been told by many psychiatrists that no child could go through what my mother put me through and not come out marked in some way.

My story is about what happens to a child who is subjected to a campaign of sustained abuse and mental torture, and how I survived.

CHAPTER 1

Beginnings

On 7 June 1963, at a house in Okehampton, Devon, I was born to my mother, Voula Sinclair, née Giorgios, in a traumatic delivery that my mother always spitefully told me had almost cost her life. She was twenty-seven years old, my father thirty-three.

My mother was Greek by birth, a war-orphan, daughter of Helena and Spiridon Giorgios. Her father had been a Nazi collaborator in the war, and both her parents had died in 1944. After the war ended, life had been difficult for my mother in Greece where mention of Spiridon Giorgios was usually followed by a curse and spit on the floor. So, in 1954, at the age of eighteen, my mother left Greece by train on a journey that brought her across Europe to Britain. For many years this was all my father knew about my mother's childhood, little realising that she harboured a most terrible secret.

My mother wasn't to be alone in this new country. Her cousin Maria, three years her senior, had made the same journey two years before, and worked as a nurse in a Cardiff hospital. Maria assured my mother that she could obtain a post as an auxiliary nurse in the Cardiff hospital, and accommodation went with the job at the nurses' quarters.

My mother had been working at the Royal Infirmary for three months when she met a young man of twenty-four who had broken his leg in a motorcycle accident. The man was my future father, Peter Sinclair.

My father came from an average middle-class family, but had been a 'high achiever' and now worked for the Foreign Office in West Germany, having graduated from Oxford University with a degree in Economics. His work was to liaise between the British authorities and the Federal German government in Bonn. However, despite his blossoming career in West Germany, my father was a frustrated man. His life's ambition had been to become an ornithologist – a studier of birds and bird life. He was a mild-mannered man, a keen studier of nature, an avid consumer of books and an enthusiastic artist. Despite his deep knowledge of post-war politics, the Middle East, and Cold War, I always thought of him as a man at odds with modern times. He had old-fashioned values, both at work and in his home life and, I think, would have been more suited to a life in the early part of the twentieth century.

In December 1954, my father, on leave at home with his parents in Cardiff, had decided to go birdwatching on his motorbike at an area of coastal marshes west of Cardiff. The weather was bitter that winter, the roads iced up at dawn. When he came to the first tight corner on a country lane the motorcycle skidded on black ice and plunged off the road into a deep ditch. My father broke his leg, and ended up in the Royal Infirmary.

My mother was shy, and my father soon became fascinated by the young nurse. She was not olive-skinned like many Greeks, her complexion was fair, her hair a rich auburn, although she soon bleached it blonde to appear more western. Due to her weak eyesight she wore glasses, which she pulled off well, and were to become one of her most distinguishing features. My father was just six years older than my mother, but looked a lot older for he already had a moustache and glasses that lent him seniority beyond his years. Genuine affection developed between my mother and father: she had a delightful laugh and a winning smile. My mother loved my father, he was what she always sought in a man – a father-figure, intelligent and capable, on whom she could rely on for emotional, financial and physical support. A romance soon blossomed, and after my father was discharged from hospital they kept in touch over the following months, meeting every time my father was on leave back in Britain.

My parents married in 1956. It was, however, a marriage that was rocky from the very start and, as he told me later, my father wondered if he had made the biggest mistake of his life. Despite knowing of his work in West Germany, it was not until after they married that my mother declared that under no circumstances would she accompany him to live in Bonn. She could not be swayed and furthermore she refused to live in Cardiff. My father tried to be understanding. Was this reluctance to follow him to Germany due to my mother's war-time experiences in occupied Greece? Did she fear Germans? he asked her. To his astonishment she was full of praise for the Germans who had occupied Greece. My mother told him that she was fixed upon her new life in Britain, and she refused to live in West Germany.

So soon after they were married, my parents rented an apartment in Clifton, a smart suburb of Bristol. Here my mother began driving lessons and passed her test in 1958. The first my father knew that she could drive was when he returned home to find my mother in possession of a white Morris Minor, and a peril on the road to anyone who got in her way.

Eventually my mother felt the itch to move again, and largely on her assertion that she wanted to live in a 'typical English town' my parents bought a large house in Okehampton in 1960.

My mother spent a lot of time on her own while my father served in West Germany, and by now she had mastered the use of English, although she still had a trace of a foreign accent. Yet bizarrely she obsessively concealed her Greek origins, and told her neighbours throughout her life that she was Swiss. She also began to use aliases; to her hairdresser she was Julie Smith, the butcher would know her as Mrs Collier, and so on. In the end it must have become a feat of memory to remember who knew her by which name. My father pondered these eccentricities very much in his last years, talking to me all through the long nights trying to pinpoint that moment in time when he realised his wife had a form of madness that was to have the most terrible repercussions. Like any slow insidious thing, what was abnormal one day becomes unremarkable a month later, and so my father told me many years later that he feared he was too easy-going, too liberal-minded. He told me he felt as if he had been the Captain of the *Titanic*, too slow to react to danger – the iceberg – until it was upon him, and too late to change course.

My early childhood was quite normal; from all accounts I was an undemanding child. My first clear memory is of holding the handle of a pushchair carrying my sister, Victoria, born just thirteen months after me in July of 1964. Two years after Victoria was born my parents decided to move to Bridgend in South Wales. It had come the time for my mother to move again, having fallen out with all her neighbours and wanting to try somewhere afresh.

My mother told my father that if we moved to Wales we'd be closer to his parents, who lived in Cardiff. However, she had no intention of actually seeing them or having them over to visit. I can clearly remember my mother, Victoria and I hiding at the back of the house in absolute silence while my mother peeped around the kitchen door waiting for my grandparents to give up ringing the bell and leave. They must have known we were at home, for my mother's car was always in the driveway. So at the age of four, I was aware that we led a strange and secretive existence.

Vicky was a precocious blue-eyed blonde with a sense of mischief that often got us into trouble. She was my sole companion in my early years as our mother avoided the neighbours and went out of her way to keep us isolated from the rest of the community. While my father was away in Bonn we never interacted with anyone outside the family. It goes without saying that my mother didn't have any friends, no one whom she could trust with her problems or ask for advice. My sister and I were part of a tight-knit group, with our mother as the leader. Every act of the day, from dawn to dusk, was organised by my mother; she even decided what games Vicky and I were to play. We were her mannequins and she the master puppeteer.

The fact is that I lived on the edge of my nerves whenever I was around my mother, which was all the time. I lived in fear of making a mistake, even of accidentally dropping something, when she would react by terrorising me. I reacted to these situations like any four-year-old child would – with frightened tears and the occasional tantrum. However, instead of trying to calm me down like a caring mother would, my mother started giving me her Valium, which quickly and conveniently sedated me and made me easier to deal with.

Every child suffers tantrums growing up as they start to assert their independence, and a loving parent would have taught their child how to cope with these. I, on the other hand, was artificially calmed down with tranquillisers. Valium affects the short-term memory, impairing a child's ability to learn. I wasn't socialised and I had no friends with whom to compare myself. From an early age, I was forced into a role that was not normal.

In 1968 my father's work finished with the authorities in

West Germany, and he came home for good, swearing that he would never again work for the British government. Something had gone badly wrong for my father in West Germany. In essence my father's job had been to receive intercepted Warsaw Pact communications from the Germans, which were then passed to the British authorities so that they could amass information about the political state behind the Iron Curtain. There was a small scandal in 1968 concerning the BND (West German Intelligence) and my father unjustly received much of the blame.

My father returned home, bitter, frustrated and unemployed. For a man of my father's experience in foreign affairs it was surprising that he had trouble in gaining immediate employment. However, early in 1969 he obtained a position at one of Cornwall's colleges of higher education, teaching foreign students and officers leaving the navy at the nearby RNAS Culdrose. This suited my parents down to the ground, for my father liked the West Country, and my mother had been itching to move again anyway.

I had started school in the September of 1968 at the age of five. Not unsurprisingly, I seemed to have become a highly strung child, prone to anxiety attacks and easy tears. I would jump at any sudden noise, and would panic if I dropped something, mostly provoked by fear of being shouted at by adults. I also suffered more tantrums – again provoked by fear of being shouted at for some transgression. I would either run and hide, throwing anything at hand to keep adults from coming near, or flop to the floor sobbing uncontrollably and hitting my head on the ground.

I also had a physical problem, which now that I had started school and was away from home became – embarrassingly – more difficult for me to cope with. Since infancy I'd had a problem holding in my pee due to a deformed sphincter muscle at the base of my bladder. This meant I had to keep going to the toilet all the time to keep my bladder empty. I also used small triangular pads of double-folded towelling to catch any leaks, which was pretty embarrassing and humiliating for me once the other children at school found out. The deformed sphincter muscle was not diagnosed until the 1980s, with the advent of new surgical technology. In 1968 the doctor could only tell my parents I was mildly incontinent, and might grow out of it as I got older.

Added to all this, I didn't immediately take to schoolwork. My first attempts at reading and arithmetic were abysmal. This may have been due to the Valium, but many young children take a while to settle into learning at school. My teacher was unsympathetic and labelled me a problem child. I was too much for her to deal with so she left me to play by myself at the back of the class, and rarely made me engage in the same activities as the other children. I soon became the target of the other children's cruel taunts and outright bullying, and I had no friends.

When my parents told me that we were moving to a mysterious place called Cornwall I was extremely happy to be getting out of school. It simply did not occur to me that the whole horrible business of education would start again after a brief respite of just a few weeks.

We moved to a three-bedroom rented house in Falmouth just before Easter 1969. As it was a holiday my parents decided that we would take our first overseas vacation together as a family, and that we would go to Greece. My mother had not been home in fifteen years. She had left Athens as a teenager to live on the far side of Europe. Now she would be returning as a thirty-three-year-old, with a lecturer husband and two children.

It wasn't a straightforward trip, not by today's standards. We travelled across Europe in my father's new Mark II Cortina, the countries growing more and more exotic the further we were from Britain. Even now I can remember my parents' unease in communist Yugoslavia. Indeed, my father drove all through the night, my mother relieving him in the daytime on truck-crowded roads. I could sense my parents' relief to leave Yugoslavia behind, this despite the fact that – during the Cold War – northern Greece, a blaze of colour and wild flowers, was heavily militarised with army observation posts seemingly on every hill.

We were to stay with my mother's Aunt Elle, who had brought her up after her parents had died. But as we drew closer to our destination it became apparent that my mother was extremely nervous about meeting her relatives for the first time in fifteen years, and she was desperate to make the best impression she could. At one point my parents had a terrible argument in a lay-by at the side of the main highway into Athens. Vicky and I sat in the back of the car watching as our parents shouted at each other in the road, she gesticulating wildly and screaming, he angry but trying to calm the situation down. Eventually my father relented simply to end the argument and to get back on the road.

It was then that I realised that my sister and I were the subject of this argument. My father would not meet my mother's eyes; they were barely on speaking terms.

My mother went to the boot of the car, rummaged in the luggage, and produced a red velvet dress, Vicky's best, and her long blonde hair was brushed into a high ponytail. She was dressed in a fitting manner to meet her great-aunt. Vicky, having been tidied, was handed over to my father, who led her away to look for flowers, while my mother dealt with me.

I found myself stripped to my underwear at the side of the road. But instead of dressing me in my best clothes as she had with Vicky, she was so paranoid that I might have an accident at Auntie Elle's house that she produced a large pad and pair of plastic over-pants, which she pulled on me. I was mortified and pleaded with her not to make me wear them. My mother lost her temper and shook me hard to make me comply. I was then dressed simply in a white T-shirt that she tucked into stretchy blue tracksuit trousers. I was very self-conscious because it was obvious that I was wearing a pad under the close-fitting trousers.

Aunt Elle's house was a huge rambling affair set in a wild garden behind high walls and stout iron gates in the affluent Athens suburb of Kifissia. It was three storeys high, all concrete, sharp angles, flat-roofed and white-painted with pale-blue woodwork. Inside it was a complex of many rooms, with a bewildering array of corridors and stairs that seemed like a maze.

When we arrived at my aunt's house we were ushered into a dim hallway, and surrounded by many relatives who chattered excitedly in Greek. My mother slipped easily into her native tongue, leaving me thoroughly confused about what was being said. My sister and I were grabbed by my aunts and uncles and hugged in order of seniority, eventually finding ourselves embraced by the redoubtable Auntie Elle. She was seventy-five, a plump kindly faced woman with henna-dyed hair, her thin arms and legs protruding from her black dress.

My mother's tone changed from excitement to sudden seriousness. She went into detail about something that left aunts and uncles tut-tutting and patting my head. I looked at my father, whose use of Greek was basic, but he knew what was being said, and I saw his face become set and angry.

Many years later my father revealed to me that my mother told them I was a difficult child who was incontinent and mentally backward, and she apologised in advance if I were a problem. Such was my mother's opinion of me.

In this house lived the extended Vlahos family. This included Auntie Elle, her daughter Sophia and husband Stamatis, who had three children of about my and Vicky's age. Auntie Elle's son George and his wife Kristina lived in the house with their two children, who were slightly older than us, and Uncle Manolis, Aunt Elle's eldest son. Everyone talked at once at high speed, and I can remember looking to my father and seeing him baffled by what was going on around us.

We were to stay with Auntie Elle for the next week. My parents, Vicky and I, were given two rooms on the top floor of the house. Auntie Elle was very religious, and at the far end of the dining room in an alcove was a shrine with an image of Christ in the Greek Orthodox tradition. On a small shelf in front burned an eternal red candle, replaced every morning by Auntie Elle. As with most Greek houses, it was dim and cool, the shutters closed to keep out the heat of the day, the air scented with the smell of spices, olives, and feta cheese. By consensus all the men took themselves off to the huge drawing room, which contained several sofas and a grand piano, to drink ouzo. The women went to the kitchen, where bright copper *brikis* produced a constant stream of strong black coffee.

That first day and evening seemed to pass quickly. Because there were so many people in the house everyone was fed in order of age. The dining room could accommodate all the family, but we seven children were fed first at 6 p.m., all seated around the big dining table. The adults, as is the custom in Greece, ate much later when we children had been sent to bed.

The following day was a whirlwind tour of Athens, with my Uncle Stamatis in the front of the car, my mother relegated to the back seat with Vicky and me. Athens was a bustling city of busy streets, markets, donkeys pulling carts, cars driven with all the ferocity of rats at the kill. The air heavy with exhaust fumes, the constant blare of car horns.

We were going to the Acropolis in the centre of the city, sitting serenely on its mount high above the chaos of crowded streets. Even after 2,000 years the marble of the Acropolis was blindingly white in the midday sun. Stamatis excitedly showed us all the highlights, as we pushed between hoards of tourists – French, British, German, even Japanese – all fanning themselves with their hats, cameras at the ready to snap some unforgettable sight.

When we returned home that afternoon it was to meet yet another relative at the family home. This was Uncle Manolis, Auntie Elle's unmarried oldest son who still lived at home. He was about forty-five years old and dressed very smartly in a merchant seaman officer's uniform with gold braid on the cuffs. He was First Officer on the Athens to Chios ferry, which crossed the Aegean twice a week. I was impressed by his uniform and very much liked this tall heavily built man with short curly hair.

That afternoon a great buffet was prepared, with many exotic delicacies laid out on the table in the dining room. Vicky and I were banished to the garden with our cousins to play while preparations were made for the feast that evening. We children played in the garden throughout the party. Uncles and aunts spilled out through the French doors on to the terrace, a glass of wine in one hand, a plate laden with food in the other.

Midway through the evening there came a great cry from my mother. Vicky and I went indoors to see what the commotion was. My mother was in the embrace of a tubby older woman wearing a very short pink dress, with long flowing dark hair. My mother chattered happily to her at great speed. Spotting Vicky and me, my mother pulled us forward, and we were introduced to this woman, who turned out to be my mother's sister, Rosa. I noted with interest how alike my mother and Rosa were. Although my mother was slim, wore glasses and was a peroxide blonde, at five feet seven inches they were the same height, and they had identical eyes, noses, and the same thin-lipped mouths.

There was an ulterior motive for my parents to drive across Europe to Greece, which even as a six-year-old I knew about from listening to their conversations. The following morning my mother and father left the house with Uncle George to visit a lawyer in the centre of the city. Vicky and I stayed behind at Auntie Elle's to play with our cousins.

It turned out that my mother had had a wealthy uncle called Andreas Giorgios – her father's elder brother – who had died the previous summer. His legacy was substantial, and to be split between his nieces and nephews, but my mother and her sister Rosa were the main beneficiaries of his will. However, in a feud that had lasted many months and was conducted with all the ferocity worthy of the Borgias, the Giorgios side of the family had fought each other most bitterly over who would get their hands on his much-desired money.

In the end it became clear that my mother and Rosa would receive about a million drachmas each (about £3,600, the equivalent of £45,000 today). However, under Greek law at the time there were strict currency regulations and my mother was not allowed to take the money out of the country. My mother returned to Auntie Elle's in a foul temper. She had come so far – in fighting her relatives and travelling across Europe – yet the money seemed as distant as if she was still in England.

Unfortunately, while my parents were seeing the lawyer, I had a small accident while playing with my cousins, and had wet myself. It was just minor, and something I felt I could deal with myself. As I spoke no Greek so couldn't explain to an adult what had happened, and because I wanted to be a self-sufficient six-year-old, I went upstairs to my room to change. The weather was warm and the plastic pants uncomfortable under my tracksuit trousers. In removing the pad and considering the situation for many minutes I took the plastic pants off, leaving them discarded on the floor next to the suitcase, and went back out into the garden, more comfortable than I had been for several days.

But then an hour later, as I was playing, disaster struck: I had another, more severe, accident and, because I had no pad, wet my trousers. Humiliated in front of my cousins, I was none the less more frightened at how my mother would react when she discovered what I had done.

It was then that my parents returned to the house. My mother saw what had happened and reacted very badly indeed. She dragged me into the drawing room, where she discovered I had taken off both the hated plastic pants and the pad. She was furious – her frustrations at the lawyer's office immediately found an outlet. In front of my aunts, uncles, and cousins peeping in through the open French doors, she stripped me of my T-shirt, trousers, and pants, leaving me bare-bottomed, dressed only in my vest.

She left me there, humiliated and sobbing in the room in front of everyone, while she stormed upstairs, returning a few minutes later with the plastic pants and a large 'night-time' pad in hand.

I wailed in anguish, looking to my father for support, but he knew better than to confront my mother when she was in one of her terrible rages. He withdrew into the garden, lighting a cigarette as he went, absolving himself of any involvement. I knew I would find no solace with him; he would not dare to create a scene with my mother before her relatives. My mother pulled the large pad and plastic pants on to me, tucking my vest into the pants and pulling them high about my waist. Then, to my dismay, I realised she had not brought any other clothes, and that I was to be left dressed only like this. My distress became very pronounced, and I sobbed anguished tears of humiliation.

I was not allowed back outside; that was the end of my playtime. I was kept indoors while my cousins, now bored, took themselves back into the garden with Vicky to play. I spent the rest of that afternoon sitting on the sofa, stripped of all dignity and feeling very alone.

At six we children were called in to eat. I was made to sit at the table with my cousins and Vicky. The other children would not look me in the eye. Immediately after I finished, my mother whisked me away to my bedroom, gave me Valium to make me sleep, and put me to bed.

The next day I was dressed again in tracksuit trousers and

T-shirt, but the damage was done. Although Vicky was accepted by our cousins, I was now an outcast. My sister had new friends for the moment, and they all refused to have anything more to do with me. My public disgrace at my mother's hands, complete with her statement to them that I was mentally 'weak', singled me out as different and stigmatised before my Greek relatives.

My mother had a more pressing problem than my comfort: she had to find some way of getting her inheritance out of Greece. She was a very cunning woman, and she was not about to be foiled by the authorities where the serious matter of money was concerned. Receiving her legacy of a million drachmas paid into a new bank account, my mother withdrew 300,000 drachmas (£1,200, about £15,000 in today's money) over the next week. This vast sum of money was then secreted in small bundles under the rear seat of my father's car.

We left Athens the next day, and headed for the Greek–Yugoslav border. It was a tense time for my parents crossing the border into Yugoslavia. If they had been caught smuggling such a large sum of money out of Greece there would have been severe repercussions, perhaps even jail. My sister and I did not understand the serious nature of what was being done as we crossed the border. Instead, seated on the most expensive back seat ever fitted to a Ford Cortina, we smiled sweetly at the border guards and we were duly waved through customs and out of the country.

A few miles beyond the border my father pulled the car off the road into a lay-by and my parents roared with laughter. Vicky and I – not understanding the joke – joined in. My mother noticeably relaxed, and then did something very odd. Getting me out of the car, she took my trousers off me and removed the plastic pants. She then let me put my trousers back on. I looked to my father who gave me an almost indiscernible shake of his head, a sign for me not to say anything. We then all got back in the car and set off on the long journey home to Britain.

CHAPTER 2

Cornwall

After an early childhood in the backwater of a small Welsh market town, the Cornish port of Falmouth in the summer of 1969 held much to interest me, with its shops, marina, docks, and Napoleonic fortress. Every weekend my parents would take Vicky and me up on to Pendennis Point, where we would stand on the cliff top and gaze down into the docks, watching the flash and spark of welders working on ships in dry-dock. Then we would continue on to Pendennis Castle for an ice cream and a game of hide-and-seek among the gorse bushes.

Following our return from Greece, in September I was sent to a local school, and the teacher, Mr Thornton, soon found the holes in my education. He made a point of meeting my parents within a fortnight of my arrival and declared to them that he was disappointed that my reading, writing, and maths skills were so poor. The junior school was very strict, and Mr Thornton known to all the boys as the strictest and least forgiving teacher there.

The house my parents rented in Falmouth was pleasant,

and within walking distance of the town centre if one took a shortcut down what is known as Jacob's Ladder – a very high set of 130 granite steps that plunges down the steep hillside from the residential sector to the town square.

One day during the autumn half term, my mother took me and Vicky shopping. We took the shortcut down Jacob's Ladder and I can remember my mother admonishing Vicky for jumping up and down the steps.

My next memory is of waking up in Falmouth Hospital, my parents sitting at my bedside. My head was bandaged and my right arm in plaster up to the shoulder. It turned out that Vicky, playing about on Jacob's Ladder, had knocked me over, sending me tumbling halfway down the steps. I was severely concussed, and my right arm broken above and below the elbow.

I spent a week in hospital, and was not sent back to the hated Mr Thornton at school for another four weeks. I had much to thank Vicky for, although Mother was furious with her, and told her off repeatedly for her carelessness. Vicky would break into noisy remorseful tears until my mother left the room, then she would grin wickedly and ask me what my arm felt like, could I feel my broken bones?

I was not sent back to school until mid-December, back to Mr Thornton, who shouted and threw pieces of chalk that sent the boys ducking as he tried to maintain order in a classroom of children determined to chatter every time his back was turned. Also I had to renew the few friendships I had made, and this was not made any easier because Mr

Thornton seemed to single me out for criticism at every opportunity. I began to dread every new school morning, and it was with some relief that the year ended with the Christmas break.

At this point my mother's mental state went into decline. She became tearful and depressed, so my father suggested she go to the doctor to see if he could give her something that would make her feel better. The doctor prescribed her Dexamphetamine and Valium. The use of amphetamine was practised in the 1960s and early 1970s, before it became clear that prescribing this medication to anyone in a fragile mental state was dangerous.

During Christmas 1969 my mother, having tired of Falmouth, demanded that we move house again. As the house was rented it did not present a problem to move quite quickly, and so in January of 1970 my parents rented a bungalow overlooking the sea at a beach village called Praa Sands, near Penzance. I was very pleased at this development, for I had begun to hate my school in Falmouth and especially Mr Thornton.

It was at Praa Sands that my mother first got into trouble with the authorities and Social Services. Since the move to Praa Sands was only intended as a temporary one, my mother did not send Vicky and me to the local school. At first this wasn't a problem. However, by late March, when Vicky and I had not been to school for over two months, a man from the education authority turned up one day to ask my mother why her children were not attending school.

Perhaps by now it goes without saying that my family lived a very strange existence, which at the time I did not see as unusual – I had nothing to compare it with after all. It was my mother's habit not to bother to get Vicky and me dressed in day clothes unless we were going out. My father had got used to this bohemian lifestyle over the years, and come to consider it normal. Thus it happened on this day, by this time mid-afternoon, that although Vicky was dressed, I was not, and wore just my pyjama top.

Confronted by a man from the authorities, my mother, put on the spot, decided to tell a lie. She pulled me forward before the man seated in the lounge and declared it was a terrible strain caring for a retarded child. To my embarrassment she told him that I was incontinent, virtually uneducable, and that it was a problem finding a place for me at a suitable school.

The man asked if that were the case why was her daughter not in school. My mother burst into remorseful tears. She assured the man that she would send Vicky to school straight away, but pointed out that finding a place for me would be difficult. She explained that my father was a lecturer, and asked if I could be educated at home. The man reluctantly accepted my mother's explanation. However, he told her that he expected Vicky to be enrolled in the local school immediately, and told her that someone would be sent from Social Services to assess whether I was in need of special education.

That evening my parents had a terrible argument. They shouted at each other while Vicky and I sat in our bedroom.

My sister and I were used to our parents' rows, our mother's volatile temper, but I can remember that this was a particularly upsetting incident. My father was furious with my mother, demanding to know why she had told such a barefaced lie that I was retarded. I cringed inwardly when I heard her scream at him that I was. Wasn't it true that at nearly seven years of age I was still wetting my pants, and so backward at school I had to have lessons apart from the other children?

My father went quiet at this and there was a long silence. I strained my ears at the bedroom door to hear what was being said. In the end I heard him say that it was true that I had problems, and I would now have to be seen by whoever was sent from Social Services.

The following week, Vicky now enrolled in school, I was due to be seen by the social worker. I could tell that my mother was very tense and short-tempered. As soon as Vicky left for school my mother made me swallow three bitter-tasting tablets.

These pills were the first part of my mother's elaborate preparations for the visit from the Social Services. It was as if my schooling and upbringing were just part of a game between her and the powers of the State, and she would not be cowed by the authorities. She went into overdrive. She put me in a large pad and plastic over-pants, then dressed me in T-shirt and tracksuit trousers.

By now I was beginning to feel really odd in a way I had never felt before. It was as if I was full of electricity and my mind darted between thoughts at high speed. I felt the need to jump about and run all the time. I was also clumsy and my tongue felt odd, leaving my speech slurred. This was the first time my mother gave me her own amphetamine tablets.

In children Dexamphetamine abuse can cause mental instability, even psychosis. Later that morning, while I was sitting on the floor, listening to whispering voices and a rushing sound in my head, the woman from Social Services came to call.

The woman and my mother sat talking together for a long time. Eventually the woman turned her attention to me. My mother made a big act of showing the woman I needed to wear a pad and plastic pants, and I was then made to sit on a chair before her. The woman asked me a range of elementary questions like my name, the day of the week, how much was five and ten, and so on. My mind felt so clogged, my speech odd, that I did not perform very well and I knew I wasn't making much sense.

Eventually the woman left, and when my mother returned to the lounge after seeing the visitor to the door she spent a long time seated on the sofa staring at me, the sunlight streaming in through the window reflecting off her glasses giving her a strange eerie quality. She did not say anything. She just stared and stared. She had declared to the authorities that I was mentally impaired. Perhaps her conscience pricked at her in some way. All I know is that I felt very unwell, and voices that made no sense whispered to me in my head. Very distressed, I broke down, sobbing quietly to myself on the floor. That seemed to snap my mother out of her trance. She got up, gave me two Valium, and put me to bed.

That spring I stayed at home, my mother teaching me reading, writing and maths. She was very short-tempered with me, slapping my hands at every mistake; in the end my fear of her exceeded that of Mr Thornton, and I concluded that education in any form was a thoroughly horrible experience. Vicky felt very unfairly treated that she now had to go to school and enviously thought that I was having an easy ride at home.

However, there were other elements of my mother's behaviour that were not very pleasant to Vicky either. During the spring my mother became obsessed with Vicky's hair, spending an hour every day brushing her hair over and over again. By the end of the ordeal Vicky was often reduced to tears.

I was treated in the opposite way. Despite the fact that Vicky was always smartly dressed and warned that she would be severely punished if she were to get untidy, I was left undressed most of the time. My mother decided I need not dress in the house, and my attire that spring was just a shirt and a pair of coloured tights. I was given no other clothing at all. At first I protested with angry tears at being dressed like an infant, but my mother shouted, shook me, and pushed me about, telling me tights were easier to wash than trousers if I were to wet them. It was the logic of a crazy person and my father, after the perfunctory initial argument, once again did not oppose her. In these early years my father still, perhaps old-fashionedly, gave my mother full control over rearing us children. He had learnt not to stand up to her, for he knew she would only take her anger out on me.

After the visit of the woman from Social Services my mother gave me two of her bitter-tasting amphetamines every day for about a fortnight. Then she gave up because the tablets made me hyperactive and I was difficult to handle. What my father revealed to me years later was that he discovered my mother had stopped taking the Dexamphetamine and Valium. What he didn't realise at the time was that she was stockpiling them against some time in the future when she might have a use for them.

As spring wore on to summer, my parents finally found a house they wanted to buy. This was no mean achievement, for they argued every time they had a viewing. My mother wanted something rural and secluded. My father felt this was unwise, yet he could not tackle my mother head on. He knew after years of marriage that she was not only unstable, but could also be very unreasonable in these circumstances.

In June of 1970, I had my seventh birthday, and shortly afterwards we visited a large bungalow on the outskirts of a town called Redruth. The house had been extended at the back, and had four bedrooms, breakfast room, a separate dining room, and large lounge. What endeared the property to my father was that it had a long drive and a very large garage with a workshop at the rear; a place to 'hide' from my mother on Saturday afternoons, in the pretence of woodwork. The redeeming feature for my mother was the fact that the property was on the edge of town on the Falmouth road, to the side and rear of the property was open countryside and there was only one neighbour.

By the time we moved to Redruth my mother had tired of having me home every day. She led a secretive life when the rest of the family were not there. Many years later, when my father at last felt able to talk, he confided to me that he never discovered what my mother had done for hours every day. The house was always clean and tidy, and she always cooked a good evening meal, but by the time he returned from work, she had often worked herself up into such a state that they would have terrible raging arguments over some trivial or implied slight, or about which my father often had no idea of the origin whatsoever. It was not a pleasant environment for any of us, sentenced as we were to screaming matches several evenings a week.

On moving to Redruth my father, much heartened with my progress in writing and arithmetic, insisted that I go to the local junior school with Vicky. Bored of my secluded life at home with my mother, I was delighted that I was finally able to go to school like a normal boy. Vicky and I were enrolled at a local junior school, and I found myself in the class of a middle-aged woman with big horse-like teeth called Mrs Craze. An unfortunate name for a teacher, and we children would make fun of it in the playground. I began to make a few friends, and my memories of that school are of long hot lunchtimes at play. Lessons were another matter, and in these I'd struggle to keep up with the other children, but so long as I wasn't getting into trouble with Mrs Craze, who seemed patient, I thought I was managing okay.

During those first months in Redruth my mother seemed to settle down, except for the increasingly frequent arguments with my father. My father would escape to his workshop, supposedly woodworking, but in reality sitting in a chair, smoking his pipe, and writing in longhand the synopses to books he planned to write. My father's literary skills had been honed over many years, and Vicky and I had got used to hearing his typewriter clacking away late into the evening.

In the autumn of 1970 my father had his first literary success, publishing a book on marketing. It was not quite the literary debut he had hoped for, but it was a beginning. My father was a prolific writer, and his first success as an author made him all the more determined to keep plugging away at his typewriter every evening and all weekend. My mother took over more responsibility for every activity in the house, from the upkeep of the home through to responsibility for us children. This was another element of closing-in, which made us all in my family inward-looking people. My father longed to stay at home and write, my mother did not want – indeed rejected – any friendships, and Vicky and I were under strict instructions never to invite any friends home. It was a world in which melodic Greek music would waft from the record player through the house all weekend. Dad would write, Mother would sit sewing elaborate dresses for Vicky, and Vicky and I played on our own.

★

The spring of 1971 became a difficult time for me in school, because once again I was falling behind the other children. I knew I was struggling to keep up, and as time went on I seemed to be falling further behind. In my frustration I also began to throw tantrums, because since February, Mother had insisted I take a bitter Dexamphetamine pill every morning to perk me up and make me more attentive. I just seemed unable to pick up the simplest maths or writing skills. Of course, I could not concentrate, and often got into trouble for letting my mind wander to the extent I did not do my work. As a result of this medication, during the spring I became highly sensitive to any conflict at home and school, becoming very agitated and crying. These disturbances were becoming problematic in school, and Mrs Craze would usher me from the class and make me sit on a chair in the corridor until I calmed down.

At home my mother continued to dress Vicky as if she was a princess whereas I was dressed in my humiliating outfit of shirt and tights. If I got upset or angry – perhaps during a squabble with Vicky over a toy – my mother would rush into the room, pin me to the floor, while screaming into my face to calm down, and would then force me to take Valium. In retrospect I don't think my behaviour differed from any other seven-year-old's, but my mother had a warped perception of me. She believed me backward and abnormal. Result: she was Draconian in her treatment of me, the slightest wrongdoing treated as a major incident.

However, by now my father had other problems to worry about than how I was being treated at home. My mother had been getting very strange during the course of the spring that year, with frequent nightmares and spontaneous tears. By April, she subsided into a sullen sort of silence. She now hardly talked, prepared meals with the minimum of grace, and took to eating on her own in the kitchen. Often she did not eat at all for days on end and was steadily losing a great deal of weight.

My father secretly went to visit our GP, Dr Greenslade. As my mother had not been to see him since the previous autumn, the doctor explained he could not say what the matter was with her. He did, however, speculate that because she was a fit and healthy woman when he had last seen her, her problem was almost certainly psychological.

Easter was a misery for everyone: my father retreated into his writing in the garage workshop, and Vicky and I played in the back garden. Mother spent all her time in her bedroom, only emerging to cook the odd meal here and there; in the end my father prepared all the meals. By the end of Easter my father decided upon his course of action. My mother would *have* to go to the doctor. But he knew that he would have to approach her very carefully, and decided to do this one Saturday afternoon. To spare us children the horrors of the row he was sure would ensue, he arranged for a neighbour to take Vicky and me to the cinema in Redruth, returning us home later that afternoon.

Years later my father was to tell me that he had a tremendous row with my mother, during which she had eventually broken down and admitted to him that she wasn't well, and agreed to see the doctor. Dr Greenslade referred her on to a psychiatrist at Falmouth's Budock Hospital.

After my mother had a long talk with the psychiatrist, she admitted the fact she was suffering terrible nightmares and flashbacks to her parents' death in 1944. The psychiatrist began to probe my mother's memories, and, with my father sitting holding her hand, she began to tell them her story, events she had never even told my father, drip by tormented drip.

She told them about the murder of her parents on 9 October 1944, in war-torn Athens, when she was just eight years old. It was a hot and dusty autumn day. She recalled the people who queued at the city's shops for the scarce supplies of food, and the drab and ragged clothes they wore. By the end of the war, Greece's situation was dire. The city was starving, and it was worse in the countryside. Everyone knew that as the Germans withdrew under pressure of the British advance in the south, a power vacuum would form, leaving the way open for ELAS (the Greek resistance) and the Communists to fight out a bitter civil war once the Germans and their puppet regime were gone. My mother's father, Spiridon Giorgios, was a leading member of ESPO, the Greek Fascist Party, who held high office in the Ministry of Interior. Of course, this meant that my mother's family was in a precarious position.

On this particular day, my mother had been with her

parents as they were driving through Athens in a chauffeur-driven car. Her father was making preparations to flee with the other leading members of the puppet regime alongside the retreating Germans. As part of the pro-Nazi administration he was terrified of what the Greek people would do to him were he to be caught by ELAS, Communists, or the British. Spiridon knew Athens would fall in a few days, and he was not planning to be present when that time came, for the Greek people would exact terrible vengeance against anyone who had collaborated with the Nazis.

Her father, my mother told the psychiatrist, had been to see the Archbishop of Athens to ask that his wife and two daughters be taken to safety by the church. They were returning home after this meeting, during which her father had pleaded with the Archbishop for his help. My mother remembered sitting in the back of the Buick with her mother and father on the way home. They rode in silence, trying not to look at the ravaged city, dusty and deserted except for a few desperate people who queued in the hope of finding a loaf of bread or a little fish. Even at the age of eight, my mother could tell that everyone was terrified, and no one could fail to notice the German soldiers who patrolled the uneasy city to keep the peace until the Nazis fled.

As the limousine had swept out into the sunlight of Omonia Square, the central hub of the commercial sector of the city, the car slowed to a crawl as the chauffeur pulled up behind an old man leading a donkey and cart. As the car pulled level with a parked truck, the peasant let go of his donkey and ran to the shelter of a nearby building. The donkey, my mother remembered, stopped and turned its soft brown eyes to gaze at the car behind it. The chauffeur blasted his horn at the donkey in an attempt to make the beast move out of the way.

Suddenly the tailgate of the covered truck dropped open and three men armed with machine-guns leapt out. They ran to the side of the car and levelled their weapons at the closed windows.

'Papa shouted at the chauffeur to drive away,' my mother recalled, 'but he froze in fear. Mama crossed herself and said "Oh my God." Then she put her hands over my eyes, as I sat between them on the back seat.

'Suddenly there was a terrible roar as three machine-guns ripped the car apart. The noise seemed to go on for ever, yet was suddenly chopped short when the three gunmen's magazines were empty. The air was heavy with the smell of gun smoke.'

In the car, my mother had miraculously survived. She opened her eyes and beheld the carnage before her.

'Papa was slumped across the seat; his face was destroyed and his right eye was missing,' my mother sobbed to the psychiatrist and my father. 'Mama lay across me, her blood turning her white silk blouse red. In the front the driver lay draped across the wheel. The smashed glass of the windows spread everywhere in spangled shards that crunched when I moved.

'I reached up to my face feeling something hot running down my cheek. When I looked at my fingers, they were covered with sticky red blood.

'I began to scream, and I couldn't stop, even when people came running to look in through the windows …'

My mother went on to tell the psychiatrist and my utterly astonished father (to whom this was a never-suspected history), that after her parents' murder, she was taken to her Auntie Elle's house. Her elder sister, Rosa, aged thirteen, stayed at home with the housekeeper, until the night Athens fell on 12 October. That night, vengeful locals forced their way into her dead parents' house, raped Rosa, and ransacked the house looking for money and jewellery.

Naturally, being the daughter of Spiridon Giorgios made life difficult for my mother and her sister in the years immediately after the war. They had gone to live with Auntie Elle. For the first time in all the years my father had known her, my mother admitted to the psychiatrist that she had a brother named Yiannis, who was two years older than she. However, he was mentally handicapped, and had been put into an asylum when he was seven years old. She never saw him again.

Unfortunately, mental illness is a stigma everywhere, but particularly so in Greece in the twentieth century, where there was little care or help available, and what was available only institutional and primitive compared with that of western Europe, unless one was prepared to pay for private care. This was particularly hard for my mother's family, for, as my father knew, Rosa was mildly schizophrenic, and periodically went out of circulation when she was admitted to a clinic. Evidently there was a difference between Yiannis and Rosa, for while Yiannis had been written off as a hopeless case and discarded into a mental asylum for the rest of his life, Rosa's schizophrenia, not a mental handicap like Yiannis's, was treated in a smart Athens clinic, her admission paid for by Auntie Elle.

My mother talked for two hours that afternoon to the psychiatrist with my father sitting to one side listening in shock to all these revelations. When she had finished the psychiatrist suggested that my mother should consider a short admission to hospital to see if they could help her. Outraged, my mother had reared up like a cobra, her hard façade back in place, and she refused his suggestion outright, declaring that under no circumstances whatsoever would she *ever* consider admission to a psychiatric unit. As my mother's condition was not severe – although it is hard to quantify what was severe under these circumstances – the psychiatrist agreed to treat my mother on an outpatient basis.

Following my mother's consultation with the psychiatrist, so astonished was my father that he telephoned my mother's cousin, Maria, who had, since her days as a nurse with my mother in the mid-1950s, married and emigrated again, this time to New Zealand. My father telephoned Maria in secret from the college, because he did not want my mother to know he was concerned and checking up on her. Maria, who had been living in Athens in 1944, confirmed the story of the assassination was true, and went on to tell my father that following the murder of her parents my mother had been so traumatised she was catatonic for six months. Maria went on to say that the discarding of Yiannis into an institution in 1941 had been particularly cruel, for the child had been quite harmless. It was just that there was such a stigma to having a mentally handicapped child in Greece that Spiridon Giorgios could not bear to have him in the house; he had been a very hard man.

Perhaps it was my mother's ethnic background, or perhaps it was a personality trait that she always possessed, but my father eventually came to believe that Spiridon's treatment of Yiannis was echoed in my mother's treatment of her own children who showed the slightest mental frailty.

CHAPTER 3

Decline

During the summer term of 1971 I began to suffer frequent disturbances in school, when I would beat my head against tables and walls. These disturbances were, I believe, in no small part due to the fact that my mother was surreptitiously forcing me to take her amphetamines, upsetting my mental equilibrium. This abnormal behaviour could not be tolerated for very long by my teacher.

In June, Mrs Craze asked my parents to visit her and the headmaster to discuss my situation. I was immediately made painfully aware I had failed abysmally, for the same day my parents were allowed to take me home early. Their attitude to me upon reaching home was harsh. With my father standing by, my mother laid into me with ferocity, screaming that I was such a problem that Mrs Craze and the headmaster had decided that I should end school two weeks early. My mother shouted that I was backward and mental, and that it had been decided I would now be assessed to see if I should be sent to a special school.

I dissolved into tears, pleading that I was sorry for failing.

No, my mother announced, if I was determined to misbehave I would not be allowed out of the house all summer, and would be sent to bed early as punishment.

Up to this point I had shared a bedroom with Vicky. However, my parents now cleaned out the small box room at the back of the house, and I would from now on sleep alone. Furthermore, I was told, if I misbehaved or had a disturbance – hit my head in frustration, shouted at Vicky, or had a tantrum – I would be locked in the room until I calmed down. And so it was that I was destined to sleep in the smallest room of the house, and be locked away if I misbehaved.

During the first weeks of August, the regime imposed upon me by my mother was very restrictive. I was not allowed out of the house, not even into the back garden, and was sent to bed exactly at 7 p.m., a full hour before Vicky. I felt a great sense of injustice at this situation.

In the second week in August my father left to teach a summer course at Cambridge University. He would be away for two weeks. I watched him pack his suitcase, knowing that without him around my mother could do exactly what she wanted to me. By that summer I was afraid of her. I had become increasingly wary of my mother that spring, but she had just been harsh. Now her expression towards me was one of loathing and hate, and I did not really know how to handle the situation, except to try to keep out of her way.

I did not have long to wait before my mother showed her

true colours. After standing at the front door the following morning to wave goodbye to my father as he drove away, Mother closed the door, grasped me firmly by the scruff of the neck, and dragged me down the back hallway where she shoved me into my room. Pleading with her not to lock me in, my only reward was a resounding slap across the face. I staggered in shock, more than actual pain. My mother had never actually hit me before, and the expression of hate on her face was something that scared me witless. The door was slammed shut, and I spent the rest of the day trapped in my room, only let out at noon for lunch. Any hope I had that this was a temporary arrangement was soon dashed, for as soon as I had finished my meal, back down the corridor I was dragged and locked in my room.

My existence continued like this for four days, allowed out only for meals and to use the toilet. On the fifth day I broke down in the corridor on the way back to my room, collapsing on the floor in floods of tears, and refusing my mother's commands to get up.

Suddenly my mother's temper snapped. She grabbed hold of me by my hair and dragged me to the dining room, where she flung me in a chair and told me to remain seated. Terrified, I stayed put. She returned a few minutes later with a handful of bits and pieces. She produced an old four-inch-wide belt, which she put around my waist, affixing the buckle behind the central panel at the back of the seat so that I could not get up. Next she took out some socks and, slapping my hands very hard and painfully, told me to make a fist. She affixed the socks tightly over my hands and arms, safety-pinning them to my pyjamas above the elbow.

'Right,' she said. 'You can stay there for the rest of the day.'

She stormed from the room, slamming the door behind her, and I found myself left alone again, this time strapped to a chair. She returned after a few minutes, and forced me to take three Valium before leaving me, closing the door behind her.

I struggled frantically in the seat trying to get loose from the belt, but slowly I felt the Valium making me light-headed and tired. And so I just sat there, for hour after hour.

Eventually at the end of the day my mother came back and let me loose, taking me into the breakfast room for tea. Then, as soon as I had finished, she dragged me from the room to lock me back in my bedroom. I had learnt that there *were* worse things than being locked in my bedroom all the time, and that my mother was quite capable of tying me to a chair if I misbehaved.

On my father's return from Cambridge I was taken to see Dr Greenslade. I stood nervously as he looked in my eyes and asked me questions. Did I ever get frightened of things I imagined? Did I hear voices when there was no one there? My mother took the lead, telling him that I had very 'odd' behaviour, was slow at school, had major disturbances and head-banging tantrums.

The doctor's diagnosis was that he believed there might be something wrong with me mentally, and told my parents he would refer me to a paediatric psychiatrist at Budock Hospital in Falmouth, the same psychiatric unit my mother had visited that April.

I will always remember the day of the appointment, for my mother made me take *four* of her bitter tablets that made me feel so odd. I was then bundled into the car and Mother, Father, and I set off for Budock Hospital.

Budock Hospital was about a thirty-minute drive from home, and by the time we arrived I was feeling really strange. Trivial things, like the pattern of the car door, seemed really important, and I spent minutes closely examining it. Also everything had an ethereal quality, like a dream, so my visit to Budock Hospital did not seem to be real to me.

I was made to sit in a chair outside a room. Eventually the door opened, and a young man asked us to come in.

The doctor undertook a cursory physical examination of me, looking into my eyes, making noises behind me and asking me to tell him which direction they had come from, and testing my reflexes. Finally he asked my parents to explain what the trouble was. My mother declared that I had uncontrollable tantrums, that I was such a problem at school the teacher did not want me in her class, and I was so backward I couldn't be taught like other children. She also lied, stating that I was prone to screaming tantrums at night, and that during these disturbances I would bang my head against the wall in a demented fashion. Despite my disorientated state I was incensed at this, for it was a lie, and I tried to interrupt, becoming very agitated and breaking down in anguished tears because no one would listen to me.

At this the doctor took hold of me by my arms and firmly sat me on a chair.

I began to sob uncontrollably because I felt so strange, ill, and nervously excited as if I wanted to run about all the time.

The doctor asked my parents if I preferred to play by myself, did I get on with other children. My mother took the lead, and with gross exaggeration told the doctor that I played odd games by myself, had no friends, was slow to learn, and often suffered tantrums when I could not get my own way.

Eventually, the doctor turned to me and asked a number of strange questions about whether I imagined things that were not real, and if I heard voices when there was no one else in the room. Feeling ill, I admitted I could hear 'whispering' voices in my head. The doctor called a nurse to sit with me in the corridor while he spoke with my parents.

Many years later I learnt from my father that the psychiatrist explained to my parents that he believed I had a serious mental condition. He was of the opinion that I was not only hyperactive, but worryingly I demonstrated the characteristics of psychosis, or, more likely, a previously undiagnosed form of mild autism. The psychiatrist told my parents that naturally this was distressing, but there had been great progress in mental care in recent years. Although autism was a serious condition, the doctor explained, my prognosis could be quite hopeful, given proper support and medication. He concluded by telling my parents that his was just a preliminary diagnosis. For a full assessment of my condition it would be necessary for me to be admitted to the primary mental hospital in Cornwall, St Lawrence's Hospital in Bodmin.

My father came out of that meeting with the doctor in complete shock. If I did suffer from a serious mental condition such as psychosis or mild autism it would explain a lot. In retrospect I think my mother was perversely satisfied that her insane plans to be rid of me were moving towards fruition.

Back at home, now with my father present to bring a modicum of sanity into the house, my mother eased up on me. I was not locked in my room any more, but she discouraged Vicky from playing with me. My mother seemed determined to keep us apart, almost as if I had some contagious disease that could spread to my sister.

Tuesday, 7 September 1971, dawned as a bright and sunny autumn day. That morning I sat as usual at the table for breakfast with Vicky and my father. My mother never sat for breakfast with the rest of the family. She was a coffee addict, and spent her time clattering pots and dishes in the kitchen while she had her fifth or even *sixth* black coffee of the morning.

After breakfast my father took me into the lounge and explained that I was going to have a few days away from home. It would not be for long, he stressed, but it was necessary for the doctors to find out what was wrong with me. This didn't worry me. All I remembered was that when I had been in Falmouth Hospital with a broken arm I had enjoyed myself playing with the toys and other children.

As Father and I left for St Lawrence's, Mum came out of the kitchen door to say goodbye. There was no affection in her farewell, her eyes behind her glasses held no emotion, much like a shark's cold mica eyes, just before it turns to take a bite out of you. I didn't try to hug her goodbye, in fact I had learnt never to try to hug my mother; she would shrink from my touch, as if I was something repellent that needed to be avoided at all costs. She disliked it when I showed any attachment or caring emotion towards her. Despite my mother's hatred of me, I suppose I still possessed at the age of eight a child's love of its mother, despite in my case accompanying fear. All I felt was sorrow, rather than hate. Hate was an emotion I never really reciprocated.

I realised as we drove through the grounds that St Lawrence's was no Falmouth Hospital; this was something entirely different. It was huge, for one thing, and while Falmouth was a general hospital, this specialised in the care of psychiatric patients. When my father parked the car before a large forbidding building, my anticipation of adventure had changed to real fear. The entrance foyer of the children's unit was all gloss paint and polished floors, and was strangely quiet, unlike the bustle of a normal hospital. I knew I didn't want to stay here.

My father opened a door, and told a woman seated behind a desk my name and explained that I had come for an assessment by Dr Smith. The woman smiled and picked up the telephone to ring someone.

For the first time I grasped my father's hand and pulled him back to ask him to take me home. He looked at me and tried in his most encouraging way to say that it was not possible. I would have to stay here until Thursday afternoon, just two nights and three days. On the third day, he promised, he would be back to collect me. It was all right, he tried to reassure me, the nurses and doctors would be very nice to me, and I would just have to do as they said until he came back.

A nurse came down the big staircase into the foyer. She smiled at me and held out her hand to take mine. I clung to my father's hand and did not let go. Despite my father telling me to be a 'big boy' and assuring me that I would not have to stay long, I began to weep. Looking at my father, the nurse suggested perhaps it would be better if he went.

My father nodded and, giving me a pat on the head, turned to go. I cried out to him not to leave me, and became very distressed. I watched Father's back as he went to the main door and let himself out, closing the door behind him. He did not look back.

The nurse picked up my bag, and proceeded to lead me up the stairs. I held back, reluctant to go, but she was very insistent and I knew that she was not about to give in to me. There was no option other than to follow her. Upstairs was a corridor with a door at the end. Taking a key out of her pocket she unlocked the door and took me on to the ward. I noticed that she locked the door behind her, and wondered why it was necessary.

The ward was a big room with a dozen children playing

with toys, yet was very institutional, with pale-green walls, yellow curtains, polished floors, and a uniformity of hospital-style furniture prevalent in psychiatric hospitals of the 1970s. She took me through to a large dormitory. The nurse, in her green uniform dress and cardigan, with a permanently fixed smile on her face, stopped at one neatly made bed and told me that this was mine for the next few days, placing my bag in a locker at the side. Then she said I could go into the other room to play with the other children.

The following morning a nurse took me off the ward, and led me downstairs to Dr Smith's office. Smiling, Dr Smith, a tall thin man with swept-back grey hair, told me to sit with him and we began to talk. I nervously looked about the sparsely furnished office, which contained a desk and a few chairs, and noticed it was identically painted in the same pale green, and had the same curtains as my ward.

Dr Smith started by asking me about my family: Did I like my sister? Did I play with her? Why did I have problems at school? and so on. Next he asked me more searching questions about my dreams. Did I ever confuse dreams with real life? Did I prefer to play by myself? Then he moved on to asking me things about what I liked on television.

After about an hour he produced papers with shapes and pictures on, asking me detailed questions about them. As we progressed the questions became much more complex, including mathematical problems. I found these increasingly hard to answer, and I do not think I made a very good job of it.

Eventually this phase of the assessment ended and Dr Smith began asking me more questions. Why did I beat my head on walls? Was it to stop panic? I didn't know the answers to some of his questions, and found myself subsiding into longer and longer periods of silence. Dr Smith did not let up, however, and persisted with rapid-fire questions on a wide range of subjects ranging from colours to friends. What were my favourite toys? Did I always play the same games with the same toys? Did I always do things in the same order? Did I understand when my sister smiled? Did I prefer cars to teddy bears? I could not follow his logic.

Feeling highly stressed and incredibly confused, I got very upset and began to cry. I just wanted him to stop his inter-rogation and let me go home. Undeterred, Dr Smith pressed on with questions that I didn't know the answers to, but he was *very* insistent and kept on and on.

Eventually – and thankfully – there was a knock on the door, and a woman put her head in. I did not catch what she said, but Dr Smith got up and went out into the corridor with her. He was soon back to tell me the test was over. The nurse would be back soon to take me to the ward.

In a few moments the nurse appeared and I was taken down the corridor to where the staircase led to the first floor. To my surprise, as we turned the corner into the foyer, there stood my mother and father. I broke free of the nurse's hand and ran over to them, upset and excited at the same time, pleading with them to take me home. The nurse rushed over and, taking hold of me firmly from behind, tried to steer me away towards the staircase. I got very upset, flopping to the floor sobbing and refusing to get up. In my deep distress I began to beat my head on the polished floor.

Many things seemed to happen at this moment. Dr Smith came to the foyer and rushed over to help the nurse prevent me from hurting myself. They both held me until another nurse appeared and took his place. The two women got me to my feet and dragged me away up the stairs. I stared over my shoulder at my parents, screaming for them to take me home, pleading and crying. We turned a corner on the stairs and they vanished from my line of sight. At this I began to scream very loudly, and the nurses hustled me down the corridor, unlocked the door and took me back on to the ward.

Once there, the nurses held me in a chair, holding my hands in my lap and pinning my legs under theirs to stop me thrashing about. All this was done while another nurse hurried into the staff office. She returned in a few moments with a glass of water and a pill. The nurses forced me to take the tablet and drink the water. The other children stared at me while I sobbed, but my need to bang my head seemed to evaporate. The nurses let go of me, and I sat in the chair utterly despondent that my parents had not intervened and weren't there to take me home.

In fact, while I sat in the chair that afternoon my parents were in deep discussion with Dr Smith. He asked them a range of searching questions about me, about my interaction with the family, my sister, did I play normally, and so on.

According to my father, who was to tell me what

happened a good ten years later, my mother took the lead in replying to Dr Smith's questions. My father felt a strong sense of uneasiness at some of my mother's answers but at this time he still deferred to my mother's judgement, and would do so for years to come. She repeatedly used demeaning phrases to describe me, saying I was 'backward'. Dr Smith asked her if I had been a slow child and how soon had I learnt to talk. My mother bluntly said she thought I was retarded, that I'd not been as quick to learn as my sister, that even now, aged eight, I was still wetting. He paid serious attention to all my mother said as she told him I was unintelligent, slow, and difficult to control, writing copious notes while she spoke. He was particularly interested when she told him she thought I did not play normally, that I seemed to live in a world of my own, that I did not interact with other children.

The following morning I was taken back downstairs to see Dr Smith. Having had such a bad experience with him the day before I was by now really frightened of him.

He pressed me with questions about whether I got confused between dreams and real life. Did I like television, and did I ever get confused by what I saw on it? Did I like my sister? Who were my friends? What games did I like? What frightened me? I couldn't understand the logic of his questions, and began to get very confused, just like the previous day. Again he presented me with a range of papers with colours, shapes, numbers and words upon them; pictures of faces with different expressions. I tried very hard to give what I thought to be the answers he wanted, convinced by now that unless I gave the correct answers I would have to stay at the hospital.

Eventually the tests finished and Dr Smith summoned a nurse to take me back to the ward. As I left he smiled, telling me that my father could take me home that afternoon. I was overjoyed at this news, and there was a bounce in my step as I went back to the ward.

Later that afternoon as I sat in the ward, a nurse came over to me and told me to follow her. She had my holdall in her hand and I realised that my father must have come for me. However, on reaching the foyer there was no one there, so the nurse told me to sit on a seat and she sat next to me. After what seemed an eternity my mother and father appeared around the corner from Dr Smith's office, with the psychiatrist accompanying them. They were talking, and stopped in the middle of the foyer to conclude their conversation.

I had a sense of foreboding because neither of my parents was smiling. Eventually a nurse appeared with two bottles of pills, which she handed to my mother. After this Dr Smith shook hands with my parents, turned and went back to his office. My parents came over, Father picked up the holdall, and we left.

It was a strange journey home. I sat in the back of the car staring out of the window and could sense the tension in the air, for my parents hardly spoke during the journey home, and then only in monosyllables, my mother's every answer terse and delivered staccato.

Once we reached home and we four were reunited at

teatime, my parents had begun to speak again, but I could tell that something was really wrong. After tea, Vicky and I were sent to the lounge to watch television, while our parents sat talking in the breakfast room. As we were used to their furious arguments it was more unnerving that there were no raised voices.

I had a growing sense of fear. What had I done? Had I failed the tests set for me by Dr Smith? Had I misbehaved by getting so upset at the hospital? And if so what were the repercussions?

All these things ran through my mind, so I sneaked down the hallway to listen outside the closed door.

I heard my father telling my mother that there was no choice now: as a result of my assessment they had to recognise that I had a serious mental condition. My mother reacted with fury in her voice, calling me 'mental'.

My father got very angry indeed at that comment, saying being cruel would not help the situation. He went on to say Dr Smith had said that with medication and support I could still live a fulfilling life; it was just I had a condition that made me different from other children. My mother grew angrier at this, and after further harsh words between them, she declared that she would look after me to the best of her ability. However, 'if' she was going to be in charge of me my father would have to 'agree here and now' that what she decided was best, otherwise arrangements would have to be made for me to go into an 'institution of some kind'.

There followed a long silence and I, terrified, strained my ear at the door. Eventually my father answered that yes, she would be in charge, and that he would defer to her about the best way to care for me.

I would now have to be sent to a special school, my mother declared, adding harshly, '*I will not allow him to interfere with Vicky's life.*'

I did not understand that, but I heard a chair leg scrape on the floor and fled back to the lounge, desperate not to be caught eavesdropping. I was too frightened to venture back down the hall to listen at the door again.

Eventually, after a long time, my parents came into the lounge and I was sent to bed. Putting me to bed, my mother produced one of the bottles given to her by Dr Smith, and gave me some tablets. It was something called Chlorpromazine, an anti-psychotic and tranquilliser, which I would now take daily through the rest of my childhood.

I was not to learn the details of Dr Smith's report to my parents for another ten years when, during a conversation with my father, long after our family had been blown to hell and back and I was old enough to understand, he told me the diagnosis. From a forty-eight-hour assessment and interviews with my parents, Dr Smith had concluded that I had a development disorder in the same spectrum as mild autism.

This diagnosis – incorrect as it would transpire – immediately exacerbated my mother's virulent hatred of me and determined the course of my life from then on.

CHAPTER 4

Downfall

Following my assessment by Dr Smith, my mother became even more aggressive and unsympathetic towards me. My father seemed powerless to stop her. Indeed, as I had heard with my own ears, my mother had blackmailed my father into giving her his support in my care at home under the threat that she would otherwise insist I be placed in an 'institution'. Under this threat my father gave in to her, and accepted her bizarre convictions of what was 'normal' and 'abnormal'. This, combined with the terrible stigma that came with being officially classified as mentally disordered, meant my mother was at last free to give full vent to her insane and obsessive hatred of me.

That September Vicky moved up a grade at school, and my father returned to lecturing at the college. I was, after my assessment at St Lawrence's, left at home until my parents made arrangements for me to attend special school.

I was totally unaware of these arrangements. I was kept at home, dressed in just shirt and tights, and received slapped legs for the slightest transgression. The only time I ever wore proper clothes was late afternoon when my mother pulled trousers on me, shoved me in the back of her Mini, and drove into Redruth to pick up Vicky from school. Slowly but surely I was beginning to fear my mother, fear her instability and rages. But worse was yet to come.

One day there was a knock on the front door and going into the hall I saw my mother take delivery of a large package. Ignoring me, she took the parcel into her bedroom and closed the door behind her. By this time my mother rarely spoke to me when we were on our own, and she often ordered things by mail order, so I was not curious. I just returned to my game in the lounge.

After a few minutes my mother summoned me to her bedroom. I saw that she had unpacked the parcel and its contents were strewn over the bed. I was curious. There seemed to be a large number of folded towels, and half a dozen pairs of pale-blue pants.

Without a word, my mother yanked my tights and pants down. She then produced a towel, a thick padded oblong with a loop of broad elastic joining both ends. Mum pulled the padded towel on me, settling the inch-wide elastic about my waist. The towelling object was a huge incontinence pad. Horrified, I pulled away from my mother, and asked her to take the pad off.

Without saying a word, but with a grimace upon her face that terrified me, she pushed me back to sit on the bed. She then grabbed the pale-blue pants off the bed, and slipped them over my feet and up my legs. They were cold and stretchy, and I suddenly realised these garments were made of rubber, with tight leak-proof cuffs at legs and waist.

The whole arrangement was horribly uncomfortable and very humiliating, and I pleaded with my mother to take them off again. She took no notice of my protests, declaring to me that she'd had enough of my incontinence problems.

'From now on,' she announced, 'these are the pad and pants you'll wear.'

She then roughly pulled the woollen tights back on me, before shoving me out of her bedroom into the hallway.

'Go on, get out of my sight, you *imbecile*!' she shrieked, shaking me, saying with anger, 'If you want to wet yourself, go ahead, I don't care any more.'

I stood crying in the hall for a few minutes. Then, despite my fear of my mother, I rebelled. Determined not to be dressed like an infant in front of everyone, I went to my cupboard in Vicky's bedroom, for I had no furniture in my box room, just a bed and chair. I pulled off the tights, removed the pad and rubber pants, and put normal pants on. Next I pulled on a pair of trousers, and headed back down the hall to the lounge to play with my toys.

Just as I passed my parents' bedroom door it opened and my mother emerged. Her eyes goggled behind her glasses, clearly shocked that I had dared to defy her. Then I saw her face set into a mask of hatred and I knew that I had made a terrible mistake. With a shriek and a stream of abuse, she dragged me by my hair back to Vicky's bedroom. There my trousers and pants were torn off me, my backside was slapped painfully a dozen times, and the pad, rubber pants and tights were pulled back on me. She seemed to be in a frenzy. Dragging me back to her bedroom, she produced three large safety pins. Pulling my tights high over my shirt, she safety-pinned them to my shirt under my armpits and between my shoulder blades at my back.

'If I can't trust you to stay dressed,' she screamed, 'then I'll treat you as the *imbecile* you are!'

Pushing me back to Vicky's bedroom, she threw all my underwear into a carrier bag. Then she dragged me out into the back garden, where she made me watch as she placed the clothes in the dustbin. I was then roughly dragged back into the house, and shoved into my room, the door slammed shut behind me and locked.

I spent the rest of the day locked in my room, with a terrible sense of fear in the pit of my stomach.

The day passed into memory, but I will always remember the shocked expression on my father's face that evening when he first saw me wearing a pad and rubber pants, with my tights safety-pinned to my shirt. However, after a few sharp words with my mother, a brief raising of voices, he did nothing.

It was at this time that my mother's psychopathic traits began to be played out on Vicky. Up to now Vicky had escaped relatively unscathed by our mother's bizarre obsessions. However, just as I became certified as mentally disordered and the focus of her hatred, so Vicky too became central to our mother's fantasy world. She became obsessed with Vicky's clothes, dressing Vicky like a living doll in elaborate velvet dresses, white knee socks, and black patent shoes. Of course, Vicky often got her hair awry, or a stain on a sock. Mother would fly into screaming rages, and Vicky was reduced to terrified tears.

My father seemed completely unable to stop the household from spiralling into my mother's insane world. He was out of the house working, some days until late giving evening classes. On Saturdays he would escape, taking Vicky with him shopping. On Sundays he would sit at his desk and clack away at his typewriter on his latest book, oblivious to the madhouse that we were all living in. I believe it was his defence mechanism, blotting out the insanity of our home by living in his own world of study, lecturing, and writing books.

One Monday morning in late September I found myself bundled into trousers and properly dressed for a change, although I was still wearing incontinence pads under my clothes. I was by now on a cocktail of tablets, not only Chlorpromazine, but also my mother's bitter Dexamphetamine, and Valium to keep me calm all day.

This morning was to be my first day at my new school. I was put in the car with Vicky, and after dropping my sister off my father drove up Redruth's steep high street to a school building behind a high wall and gates with a sign proclaiming it to be Curnow Special School. Curnow School was a typically late-Victorian Cornish building, granite with high arched windows and echoing corridors.

Here he handed me over to a woman who took me into

a small classroom of ten children. It was a pleasant, sunny room with tables and chairs, pots with crayons on each table, and children's pictures hung on the walls. It was only when I looked a little closer that I discovered that this was no normal school. To begin with there were two teachers to this class of ten boys, and the pupils were clearly at differing places on the mental-health spectrum; two of the boys had Down's syndrome.

It wasn't long before I found myself shamed before my new friends and teacher. On Thursday afternoons my class had use of the hall for the games lesson. The first I knew of this was that day after lunch when the teacher told all the boys to take their clothes off and put on their T-shirts and shorts if they had them. At first I pleaded with the teacher, Mrs Grey, not to make me undress because I had not brought any PE clothes with me.

The other children had by now taken their clothes off. Some had changed into gym clothes, and half were standing barefoot in just vest and pants. Mortified, I explained to my teacher I had 'problems' and my mother made me wear a pad and special pants. Mrs Grey told me that she knew I wore a pad, and added that some of the other children had problems too, but they had undressed.

She proceeded to 'help' me undress. In moments I was left standing barefoot in just vest and rubber pants. I saw her stunned expression at the sight of what I was wearing, but she said nothing. I had often felt very humiliated by my mother's treatment of me, but that afternoon was particularly bad for me as I played with the other boys, shown up before my teacher and new friends. I realised that I would have to think of something drastic by next week if this was not to happen again.

The following week I came up with a solution. Despite the fact that my mother sorted out a T-shirt and shorts for me to wear on Thursday afternoons, I would, I decided, stop wearing the pad and appalling rubber pants.

I sneaked into Vicky's bedroom one evening and found my swimming trunks. Victorious, I hid them under my bed. Thursday arrived and before departing for school I dashed to my room, yanked off the hated rubbers and pad, and threw them under my mattress before re-dressing in the trunks and trousers.

I went to school happy that day. I had accomplished a minor victory over my mother, and I decided that from now on I would take my care into my own hands. I could sneakily change my underwear without my mother ever knowing.

It was a small victory, however, and short-lived. I was still slightly incontinent due to my deformed sphincter muscle. My only defence was to keep going to the loo to keep my bladder empty.

About mid-morning on that fateful Thursday I suddenly had the urge to pee, but before I could ask to go to the toilet I had an accident. I was prone to minor accidents and this I could have coped with. But this wasn't minor, and my trousers were soaked. Tearfully I went to Mrs Grey to explain that I'd had an accident.

There was nothing for it, Mrs Grey declared, I would

have to go home, and she telephoned my mother to come to collect me.

I was doubly unfortunate that day, for my mother had already discovered what I had done. Making my bed, she had found the incontinence wear hidden under the mattress.

My mother was furious when she came to collect me, and I knew I had made a terrible mistake when I saw her expression. She did not speak to me all the way home and, seated in the back of her Mini, I was terrified of what would happen.

It was not until she slammed the front door behind us that she flew into an insane rage, screaming at me and shaking me very hard. I found myself dragged into the kitchen where she stripped me naked, throwing all my clothes into the washing machine. I was then put over a chair and my backside slapped hard a good twenty times. She left me huddled up naked on the breakfast-room floor sobbing. When she returned I was yanked off the floor and re-dressed in the pad and rubbers and an old shirt. Dragging me by my hair, she took me down the back corridor and shoved me into my bedroom. Holding me by my hair she aimed three resounding slaps across my face before flinging me on to the bed and locking my door.

I lay on the bed, desolate, and sobbed my heart out, terrified of my mother, and in full realisation that I led a dreadful life that I had no control over.

That same day my mother telephoned Dr Smith, and told him she could not cope with me. She lied to him, claiming I was impossible to manage, that I was behaving bizarrely by taking my clothes off at inappropriate times.

Dr Smith listened to my mother's exaggerations, listened as she told him about my difficult nature, my frequent disturbances and tantrums, and now stripping to remove my incontinence wear, after which I was wetting myself. Dr Smith told her that mentally disordered children occasionally had this odd behaviour; it was known as a 'strip and soil' trait. He told my mother that I should be prevented from doing this, and gave her the details of a company that manufactured special anti-strip clothing for mentally disturbed children.

For a fortnight after the accident I had at school, an uneasy truce existed between my mother and me, and I believed that she had forgiven me. However, I was mistaken. She was merely biding her time.

Picked up from school on a Friday afternoon by my mother, I sat quietly in the back of her Mini while we waited outside the junior school for Vicky. Vicky soon appeared among a gaggle of children, immaculately dressed as always, and climbed into the car to sit beside my mother in the front. I resented the fact that Vicky, a year younger than me, was allowed to sit in the front of my parents' cars, while I was always made to sit in the back.

At home my mother immediately took me to my bedroom, where she made me take my school clothes off, stripping me down to my underwear. She then grasped my arm and bundled me back down the long front hall to her bedroom.

In my parents' room I noticed that there were two large brown paper parcels on the bed. I stood still while my mother delved into one of the packages and pulled something out.

At first I thought it was a pair of trousers, until she unfolded it and I saw that it was a blue bri-nylon jumpsuit: an all-in-one with stirruped feet, no sleeves and zipped up at the back. I was made to put it on. It was close-fitting and made of the same stretchy material as my tracksuit trousers. Turning me around she pushed my arms through the sleeve holes, then did up the zip and fiddled at the top with a small flap of cloth that secured the zipper with a tight-fitting button. She pulled me around to face her. There was a look of satisfaction on her face. My mother now tore open the package and I saw that it held five more of these jumpsuits, three red and two blue.

I put my hands over my shoulders behind my neck to try to reach the zipper, and found with the tips of my fingers a very tight-fitting rubber button that needed to be undone before I could unzip the jumpsuit.

'Stop it!' my mother snapped, slapping my hands and pushing them away.

I put my hands back down, pleading with her that I couldn't wear a jumpsuit because it was horrible and made me look different.

'I don't care,' my mother snapped back at me. 'If you behave like you're mental then this is what you'll wear from now on. I won't have you stripping.'

I replied, on the edge of tears, that I didn't 'strip'; my mother took no notice. She just gave me a hard shake and told me to be quiet.

Turning me around, she undid the zip and took the jumpsuit off me. I was relieved, thinking this was the end of the ordeal. I had learnt through bitter experience to fear my mother when she was like this. In the mood she was in at the moment, she did not treat me – or Vicky – as persons. At these times she treated her children as objects that *had* to be compliant, otherwise she could fly into a most terrifying and violent rage. I subsided into frightened silence, and just stood there as the jumpsuit was discarded on the bed with the other garments.

Next she turned her attention to the other package and tore that one open too. On the duvet were six pale-green garments. My mother picked one up and let it fall open. It was a complete all-in-one with arms and legs like a pair of long-johns, and I watched as she, with some difficulty, undid the six large tight-fitting rubber buttons down the back. It was another humiliating thing that I had to wear, and I shrank away from her as she approached me.

'Come here!' she ordered, and I, too afraid of her to disobey, went to her.

She pushed me to sit on the bed while she got my legs into the all-in-one, then yanked me to my feet and forced my arms down the sleeves.

I looked down at the long-johns as she struggled with the rubber buttons at the back. It was, like the jumpsuit, close-fitting. It was elasticated at the ankles and wrists, and the neckline had an inch-wide hem of tough yellow duck-cotton. This tough hem also ran down the back, and I could tell that it would take considerable strength in the fingers to twist the six rubber buttons through the very tight eyes. Eventually, my mother managed to do up the buttons. Pulling me round to inspect the garment, she pulled and shoved me, while she fingered the neckline and pinched under my arms to see if I could get it off.

'Please,' I pleaded with my mother. 'Don't make me wear this. I won't take the pad off again, I promise, and I won't ever undress.'

'I don't care,' my mother snapped. 'This is what you'll wear from now on. I've had enough of you, and I don't care about you any more.'

And with that she grabbed me roughly by the scruff of the neck, opened the bedroom door, and shoved me out into the hall. She turned on her heel and went back into her room, slamming the door behind her, and left me standing there in the hall not knowing what to do next.

When my father returned home that evening, and I had struggled without success to take the horrible long-johns off, I pleaded in tears to him not to be made to wear an all-in-one.

His face, when he saw me in the horrible all-in-one, was full of shock and concern, and he went to the kitchen to seek my mother out. I heard raised voices from the back of the house, but again he did nothing, and I was left dressed in this humiliating garment. A short while later Vicky and I were called to tea. I sat self-consciously at the table, very aware that my entire family were well dressed and immaculate, and I was now attired as if I were severely mentally disordered, in the tight-fitting all-in-one with a very evident pad underneath. It was more than I could bear, and, filled with utter humiliation, I began to cry. Of course, this didn't help my situation. My mother dragged me roughly from the table to the bathroom, where she threatened me, stating that if I didn't behave she would lock me in my room, where I would stay all weekend.

I spent the whole of that weekend dressed only in the all-in-one, night and day, not allowed out of the house, and made acutely aware that Vicky was the 'clever' child who was dressed immaculately and allowed to go shopping with my father when he went out on Saturday. I was at the opposite end of the spectrum, kept in humiliating clothes and treated as if I were a very mentally disturbed child.

On my first day at school wearing just a red jumpsuit and patterned shirt, my mother met with Mrs Grey. She told her that both she and my psychiatrist, Dr Smith, had decided that because of my tendency to 'undress' (which was not true) it was now necessary for me to wear anti-strip clothing. Mrs Grey sympathised with my mother, and from then on the classroom assistant escorted me to the toilet to undo the jumpsuit.

As Christmas approached, I began to become less and less mentally stable. By this time I was on a daily dose of the anti-psychotic Chlorpromazine, prescribed for me by Dr Smith, plus one or two Valium to keep me quiet. I would now become so disturbed that I would end up beating my head against walls and floors, during which time I would have to be pinned down on the floor to stop me hurting myself. Clearly my state of mind was extremely fragile. However, unknown to Dr Smith or my father, my mother was by now forcing me to take two, sometimes even three, Dexamphetamine tablets a day, and by December I had been taking this dangerous drug for nearly a year.

Christmas of 1971 came, and at my father's insistence I was dressed in normal clothes for Christmas Day, so he could photograph me and Vicky opening our presents. On Boxing Day, back in an all-in-one, I squabbled with Vicky. It was just the sort of argument that most normal siblings have occasionally, but my parents thought I was throwing a tantrum. Instantly they pounced on me, held me down on the floor and forced me to take two Valium tablets to calm me down. After that I spent the rest of the afternoon in a sedated state, and was put to bed early at 6 p.m., after which Vicky and my parents continued their festivities without me.

In January 1972, having returned to school after Christmas, Mrs Grey asked my father to visit her. Having had many years' experience in teaching mentally disordered and impaired children, she was concerned about my mental state. My medication regime had upset my mental state; this, combined with head-banging tantrums, frequent easy tears and perpetual agitation, made Mrs Grey think that I was becoming severely mentally disordered. She told my father that I appeared to be noticeably declining, and was increasingly prone to severe episodes in which I would mercilessly beat my head against tables, walls or floor. She remarked that at these times I was verging on the point of being beyond the care of Curnow Special School.

As a result of this conversation with Mrs Grey, my parents took me to see Dr Smith in late January, and he, after examining me and discussing my case with them, dramatically raised the level of Chlorpromazine I was to be given, trebling the dosage and sanctioning greater use of Valium whenever I was agitated or disturbed.

In the first week this higher dosage of Chlorpromazine left me very sedated and lethargic all day long. 'Like a zombie', according to my father. Kept at home for the first week of this increased medication and left in those hideous long-johns all day, I was so sedated that I could hardly eat my meals, could not play, and spent the entire day just slumped on the sofa, half-awake in a nightmare world where – my mind clogged – I felt too 'heavy' to move. My condition suited my mother. I was pliable; she could put me in a chair and I stayed there; I hardly talked – and even then only in monosyllables: I was no trouble at all to control.

When I returned to Curnow School in February, a fortnight after Mrs Grey had last seen me, she was so concerned at how my mental state had deteriorated that she told my father when he came to collect me that I was now so sedated I was almost uneducable. My father telephoned Dr Smith to ask if the medication could be reduced. He was told to persevere because I would eventually acclimatise to this higher level of Chlorpromazine. Dr Smith emphasised to my father that he thought I showed signs of an early onset psychotic syndrome, common in autistic children, and that this raised level of medication was necessary to control the condition.

My father was yet to realise in February 1972 that Dr Smith's words would turn out to be prophetic. It was not that I was really autistic, or indeed psychotic, at least not then. However, my mother's continued mistreatment and meddling with my medication was enough to cause any child's mental state to collapse, and by now my mental state was becoming increasingly precarious.

CHAPTER 5

Psychotic

Shortly before Easter 1972, my parents decided to buy a Bedford motorhome. This meant that my father reluctantly agreed to part with his cherished Cortina, because my mother told him that as a family we would from now on have enjoyable camping holidays together. This sounded great to my father, and the loss of the Cortina was an acceptable trade-off.

However, my hopes for a holiday that Easter were dashed within hours of our acquiring the Bedford, and I think that in his own way too my father had been deceived by my mother.

The same afternoon that my father brought the Bedford home, my parents had a terrible argument during which my mother told him that under no circumstances was she willing to take me on holiday with them. She said that because I was a problem child with a mental condition and incontinence problems and required constant supervision, she was not prepared to look after me in the confined space of a motorhome.

Within a day or two my mother telephoned Dr Smith to ask him what were the requirements for me to be admitted to institutional care. Dr Smith told her that I was not mentally disordered enough to warrant admission to care. However, if my mental state deteriorated that was another matter. In an attempt to placate my mother, he told her that as a child certified under the Mental Health Act as autistic I was now eligible for periods of respite care, and that there was a suitable children's unit in Camborne.

And so it was that during Easter 1972 I found myself taken in the Bedford to a big house in Camborne, where, holding me roughly by my arm and carrying a large plastic carrier bag of clothes in her other hand, my mother handed me over to strangers. It was a traumatic ordeal for me and I got very distressed, because I had, until that morning, no idea that I was to be put in a care home for ten days.

The care home was a large house, but institutional with cold lino floors, gloss-painted walls, and a pervasive smell of disinfectant. I was appalled and embarrassed on my arrival, when my mother made a special point of telling the woman in charge that because I was incontinent, and disordered and autistic with the habit of stripping, my psychiatrist and she had decided I needed to wear anti-strip clothes day and night. My mother seemed to take a perverse satisfaction in humiliating me and making an example of me at every given opportunity.

It has occurred to me since that perhaps she thought that by increasing the pressure on me, in addition to meddling with my medication, she could drive me off my head, in which case Dr Smith would agree to place me in institutional care, and then she could be rid of me for good. My placement at this care home for ten days would be the first opportunity she had to experience what life would be like if my family consisted of just her, my father, and Vicky, and I think she found the prospect pleasing.

It turned out the home was not an unpleasant place. Everyone on the staff was very kind, but all of the children there had severe mental-health problems, and it was not possible to play or to talk to them in any but the simplest of ways.

I felt very lonely among the playroom full of 'odd' children. The staff just made sure everyone stayed calm, doled out medication, provided meals, and made sure everyone was in bed at 7 p.m. To my mortification every evening I found myself singled out when a woman publicly changed my pad and rubbers in front of the other children, and put me into my all-in-one after my bath, before putting me to bed. Even the most impaired children here didn't have to wear anti-strip clothes, and I had a good weep at my predicament that first evening.

Eventually, after ten days, my mother appeared in the playroom and called to me. To my relief I found myself taken outside to her Mini. My ordeal was over, and I was pleased – grateful – just to go home. On my arriving home, Vicky came bounding up the hallway and hugged me. To my indignation she now announced she'd had a great holiday with my parents in France, and sleeping in the motorhome was wonderful.

The realisation that I had been dumped in a home for

mental children, and excluded from the family holiday, left me angry and distraught. I never forgot what had happened, and the horrible injustice of it all.

The summer term of 1972 was short and soon the holidays were upon us. I now stayed at home with Vicky, and spent all day in the large back garden, where we'd cycle around the perimeter for hour after hour.

My mother was in a better state of mind at this time, and this meant we children had an easier time of it. It turned out that she was pregnant, and both Vicky and I were intrigued by the fact that in the New Year we would have a new baby sister or brother in the family.

At the beginning of August my father began to prepare to go to Cambridge for his annual course. I was worried about this because when he had gone away in the previous summer I had spent most of the fortnight locked in my room. However, I also hoped that this wouldn't be the case this time. Surely, I thought to myself, now that my mother was being easier on me she would not do that again. But of course the way she behaved towards me was quite different when my father was not present.

The day of my father's departure for Cambridge came. I watched him back the Bedford out of the driveway and drive away. Vicky, Mother and I stood waving to him as he vanished down the road, and then we went indoors.

On closing the front door, my mother grasped me, and told me that I was not allowed out of the house while my father was away. I was to stay indoors.

Distraught at being told I could no longer go out to play on my bike with Vicky, I pleaded with my mother not to make me stay indoors. Holding my shoulders, she shook me and told me to behave, otherwise she would that very moment put me in my room.

I was now continually left in my all-in-one and not dressed in day clothes at all. My mother also began to dramatically meddle with my medication, which of course directly affected my mental state. On getting me up in the morning she gave me too much Chlorpromazine, which made me lethargic and easier to manage. At lunchtime she gave me several Dexamphetamine tablets to 'perk me up', but then gave me Valium in the afternoon to calm me down again.

During the time my father was in Cambridge something happened which was to have devastating repercussions on my mental state; in fact it contributed to sending me over the edge into a state of true childhood psychosis.

One lunchtime my mother was preparing a meal of fish fingers. Vicky and I were playing tag in the breakfast room. Somehow I found myself in the kitchen and I accidentally bumped into my mother, knocking the frying pan from her hand. It clattered to the floor, the fish fingers tumbled everywhere and scalding fat spilled on to my mother's foot. She let out a scream. Turning the cooker off, she fled the kitchen in tears and ran to her bedroom. Vicky and I looked at each other in silence.

My mother eventually returned half an hour later in a terrible rage. On her bare foot was a bandage, and she was limping. I knew I had inadvertently hurt her, and I knew by the expression on her face that I was in for it. I was terrified of her and she knew it. She grabbed me, screaming that I would be punished for misbehaving and, holding me painfully by my arms, she shook me and shook me. Shouting that she had had enough of my mental behaviour, that she hated me, and that mental children who were dangerous need to be locked up, she declared that I would be strapped to a chair to teach me to behave.

I was pushed to the floor, and Vicky was ordered to make sure I didn't get up. I was absolutely terrified by now, and the threat that I would be strapped to a chair brought back horrific memories of the previous summer when she had actually done that to me.

As soon as my mother left the room I scrambled to my feet and ran out of the back door into the garden. I ran over to the garden gate and fled down the driveway. Despite the fact that I was dressed only in slippers and an all-in-one in the middle of a hot summer's day, I ran out into the road and, terror taking reason from my nine-year-old mind, fled down the pavement as fast as I could go.

After about quarter of a mile I came to a set of traffic lights. Beyond this was Clifton Road, a street of smart big houses. It occurred to me that I should go to Dr Greenslade, whose surgery was in Clifton Road. He was the only adult I knew who might help me.

I only got about a hundred yards down Clifton Road when I saw a police car pull up ahead of me and two policemen got out. I dashed across the road, narrowly missing a passing car, which blared its horn. The two policemen ran across the road to cut me off. Cornering me against a wall, they approached me, holding their hands out in placating fashion, trying to calm me down. By now I was sobbing hysterically. The policemen took hold of me, and put me into the back of the car, one of the men seated next to me. Sobbing and pleading to be taken to Dr Greenslade, I found myself taken home. My mother had telephoned the police as soon as I ran away.

The police car pulled up outside the house and the two policemen took me to the front door, which was opened by my mother, who asked them to bring me inside. I listened between sobs as my mother told the two men that I was a disturbed, mentally ill child. She produced two Valium tablets and, with the policemen still holding me, made me take them. All three adults then forced me to sit on the floor, and held me there as they continued to talk about me. Eventually, the tablets began to have an effect and I calmed down; the policemen then let go of me and left.

On closing the front door behind her, my mother turned to me with a look of complete hatred on her face. She grabbed me, slapped me with a resounding crack across the face, and dragged me stumbling down the hall to the dining room. Opening the door, I immediately saw the chair already prepared in the middle of the room, the wide belt draped over the back.

I screamed and pleaded not to be put in the chair, but my mother took no notice and, after a brief struggle, forced me into it. The wide belt was placed around my waist and secured at the back. She then went to the table, where I now noticed there was a collection of bandages. To my horror she wound a bandage tightly six times about each wrist, tied it off, then tied it to the arms of the chair. She did the same to my ankles, tying them to the chair legs. Within minutes I was completely immobilised, securely strapped and tied to the chair. Next, the curtains were drawn, and she left, slamming the door behind her.

I continued to sob, screaming to be let loose. Suddenly the door flew open, and my mother stood there with a towel in her hand. She came over to me as I sat struggling in the chair and sobbing. She placed the folded towel firmly over my face and held it tightly in place, smothering my cries. Shouting in my ear, she screamed that if I didn't stop making a noise she would gag me. Terrified, I subsided into silence.

'I hate you!' she shouted angrily. 'This is where you'll stay.'

She stalked from the room, slamming the door behind her.

I remained in the chair for the rest of the afternoon until teatime, when my mother returned with a bowl of baked beans, and untied the bandages from the chair arms to let me eat my meal. As soon as I finished my wrists were securely retied to the chair arms.

I was sobbing again by now, pleading with my mother to let me loose, that I needed the toilet. I was sorry, I cried, I hadn't meant to hurt her or run away. All this had no effect on my mother. She ignored me completely and left the room, slamming the door behind her. My backside was completely numb from sitting for hours, and my bowels ached dreadfully for I desperately needed the toilet.

In the evening my mother returned with a cup of water and my medication of Chlorpromazine, plus several Valium tablets. Forced to take them, I sobbed to her to let me loose; even being locked in my room was better than this.

'I've had enough of you,' she shrieked. 'I absolutely hate you, hate you, *hate you*! If you're an *imbecile* that can't be trusted to behave, this is where you'll stay.'

I was sobbing dreadfully now, not only because I was terrified of her, but also because my backside ached appallingly from sitting for hour after hour and from the strain of trying to hold in my stools. Distraught, I pleaded with her to let me go to the toilet.

She responded that she didn't care if I needed the toilet. I would stay in the chair as punishment until I learned how to behave. She'd had enough of looking after a mental child.

'You *imbecile*!' she shrieked into my face, her nose an inch from mine. Then she slapped my face hard before stalking from the room and slamming the door behind her.

Really terrified now, I struggled dreadfully in the chair, but it was no use. At long last I could not hold on any longer and, sobbing, I soiled myself.

Eventually, the medication made me fall asleep. I awoke in the pitch dark and to a house in complete silence.

In my fear and terrible discomfort, for I had an awful prickling numbness in my arms and legs through lack of circulation, I now began to cry, calling out to be let loose. I must have been sobbing and calling out for twenty minutes before the door was suddenly flung open and the light switched on, momentarily dazzling me.

My mother stood there in her dressing gown, holding a towel in her hand. I squirmed and rolled my head back and forth as she struggled to hold me. Then she held me by my hair and placed the folded towel firmly over my face, smothering my cries. It was terrifying for I could hardly breathe.

'I hate you, *hate you*!' she screamed. 'I wish you were *dead*! If you don't shut up I'll gag you!'

I subsided into a terrified silence and, after what seemed an eternity, she took the towel off my face and I could breathe again.

'I've had enough of you!' she shouted. 'I *hate* you! Mental children who're dangerous should be locked away!'

Once more I sobbed that I was sorry for hurting her, sorry for running away, and pleaded to her to let me go to the toilet.

My mother, her face almost touching mine, my head held by my hair and her hand clasped over my mouth, screamed into my face to be quiet.

'You'll stay in this chair, you stupid little *imbecile*!' she shrieked. 'If you want the toilet you're in a nappy so go ahead…'

And with that she slapped me hard across the face and left, turning off the light behind her and slamming the door, leaving me in complete darkness.

I spent the rest of that night sobbing. It was worse than a

nightmare and I was agonisingly uncomfortable. My hands, arms, legs, and feet were completely numb, my behind and bowels ached abominably.

The next day my ordeal continued. My mother kept me strapped to the chair. I was brought a drink in the morning, my hands set free for lunch and tea, and retied as soon as I finished. I was too terrified to call out, and, after thirty-six hours strapped to the chair, I was in a truly horrific state.

In the late evening my mother eventually came with a pair of scissors and cut the bandages, freeing my hands and feet. She then undid the belt and I fell from the chair to sprawl on the floor. I was numb all over and in agony through lack of circulation. I couldn't even crawl, let alone stand up. I just lay on the floor sobbing in pain, my arms and legs useless and tingling, my hands and feet throbbing as the circulation was gradually restored. My mother's response was to grab the back of my all-in-one and physically drag me across the floor, down the long hall and into the bathroom, where she stripped me and gave me a bath. After this, with not a word spoken to me, I was re-dressed in clean pad, rubbers, and all-in-one, forced to take a handful of tablets, and then locked in my room. I collapsed on my bed utterly exhausted by my horrific ordeal.

I was now truly terrified of my mother. A boundary had been crossed, and as I lay on my bed what echoed in my mind over and over again was my mother's voice screaming that she *hated* me, and calling me an *imbecile*. These voices were the first hints of a psychosis that would lurch over into auditory hallucinations and would soon send me over the brink into a true and terrible mental illness.

With my father's return home, the household returned to a sort of normality.

My mother expressed her hatred of me to my father, telling him that I had caused the accident in the kitchen that had burnt her foot. She also told my father about my running away in just my all-in-one, that she needed to call the police to get me back, and declared that I was truly mentally disturbed. There was no mention of the punishment she had inflicted on me, and I was too terrified of her to tell my father what she had done to me.

I would say that my decline into a state of actual psychosis began about October 1972. In my case, the descent into psychotic illness was a slow, insidious thing, and definitely had its origins in my mother's mistreatment of me in the summer. I began to have problems discriminating between what was a dream and what had actually happened. People with psychosis have problems discerning what is reality and can descend into their own make-believe world. Psychosis is a loss of touch with the real world, often accompanied by hallucinations, both visual and auditory, a state in which the mind becomes unbalanced and is no longer able to tell reality from fiction.

By November of 1972, at the age of nine and a half, I began to have nightmares in which my mother was chasing me, and I could not work out whether this had happened or not. On one occasion I dreamt that my grandparents had come to visit, and wouldn't believe my father when he told me they were not present, searching the house and becoming completely distraught, until in the end my parents had to give me Valium to calm me down. I also began to have what I can only describe as powerful dreams while I was awake, and heard voices shouting at me. Lacking insight to realise it was just my own mind becoming ill, I began to get very confused.

Sometimes I became so frantic I'd beat my head mercilessly against walls and floors to stop the voices in my head. Believing my dreams to be real, I would wake up screaming in the middle of the night, and I became very confused by things I saw on the television. Many children get frightened of something they see on the television, but in my mentally weakened state I actually believed these things to be real, becoming terrified for days on end.

Concerned at my decline, in December my father took me to see Dr Smith. After an examination, during which Dr Smith asked me a series of curious questions about my imagination, and asked me whether I heard voices in my head, I broke down and announced that my mother hated me, and that she was shouting at me even when she was not there, during school or in the middle of the night.

Dr Smith reached for the phone and called for a nurse to sit with me in the corridor while he talked to my father. Many years later my father told me that Dr Smith explained that I exhibited symptoms of a psychotic illness. It was a very serious mental condition. He increased the dosage of Chlorpromazine, but there really was no other treatment other than time and patience. I would have to be kept quiet at home, not over-stimulated, and given a lot of care.

And so it was that I found myself kept at home, and heavily medicated every day, throughout December. Everything possible was done to keep me quiet. I was given a lot of Chlorpromazine and Valium, permitted to watch only the simplest children's programmes on television with Vicky at teatime, before going to bed at six o' clock.

By now I was far from well. I couldn't hold on to my thoughts, my memory was shot to pieces, and I became very confused. I was also hallucinating a voice that told me I was stupid and that I should hurt myself.

After Christmas, my father went back to his job and my sister returned to school. By this time my mother was very pregnant indeed, and could not cope with me at all. I was now in a state of complete mental collapse, and not only did my mother not want to cope with me, but I suspect she physically and psychologically could not cope with the consequences of the damage she had inflicted on me over a period of years.

Early in January my father took me back to see Dr Smith. The prognosis was not good. Dr Smith was extremely concerned at my decline, which he now declared was clearly severe psychosis. My father was horrified by this diagnosis, especially when Dr Smith declared that although his original assessment of mild autism had certainly been correct, perhaps I had always had a lurking form of psychosis.

From now on I spent all my time at home dosed up on Chlorpromazine, and given Valium when I became frantic.

My parents now took to locking the front and back doors at all times in case it came into my mind to wander off. On the occasions I became distraught, either through thought disturbances (such as when I became convinced that there were daleks waiting for me in the bathroom), or by hallucinations, and began sobbing uncontrollably, my mother would bundle me into my room and lock the door. I would scream and beat my hands against the door, but she never came back.

In the way of psychosis, I began to lose the distinction between night and day. I would keep my father awake all night long as he tried to calm me down, which was almost impossible when I was hallucinating. It was truly a psychotic illness in its most virulent form. My memory of that time is very sketchy, but I can still vividly recall terrifying visual hallucinations: my horror at seeing things with sharp teeth snapping at me coming out of the wall; the snake-like things darting about on the periphery of my vision that made me scream and crouch in the corner.

In February 1973 my mother gave birth to a baby girl, whom my parents named Ingrid. Ingrid was, against medical advice and my father's wishes, born at home.

With my decline into a state of severe psychosis my mother began to hate me with an unremitting fervour. Up to mid-January 1973, I had at least been cognitive every now and again. After the birth of Ingrid I descended into a psychotic world of my own, plagued by terrifying hallucinations that left me without reason. By February of 1973 there was very little that could be done for me, except sedate me all the time to keep me as quiet as possible.

Because of my mental state at the time I do not remember much about this period and my memory is limited. I recall a hazy world where I was locked in my room every night, then all day, too. In effect I became a psychologically damaged prisoner of my mother, locked away in my room at the back of the house.

Combined with the extra strain of caring for a newborn, my parents found they could not look after me in the terrible state that I was in. A fortnight after Ingrid was born, steps were taken to place me as an in-patient in the Children's Unit of St Lawrence's Mental Hospital. One day, long in the future, my father would tell me that on 20 February 1973, he called Dr Greenslade to the house to examine me. The doctor found me in a completely psychotic state, extremely agitated and not talking any sense at all. He called for an ambulance, and it was by this means that I left Redruth and my parents, and was admitted as an in-patient at St Lawrence's Hospital.

I do not remember my first weeks at St Lawrence's. Indeed, I still only recall fragments of much of the second month. However, as my recovery progressed under careful medication and care, I slowly began to recover my mental equilibrium, and became less psychotic. It was like waking up from a very deep sleep in which you've been tormented by traumatic nightmares. I was completely psychotic for about six weeks, and only began to recover in April. February and March of 1973 are almost completely lost to me.

My early memories of life at St Lawrence's seem to mainly consist of huddling up on the floor of the children's ward, motionless and feeling 'spaced out'. To begin with I didn't know where I was. My mental state gradually improved to the point where I began to recognise the fact that I was wearing a dressing gown, and that I was on a ward of twelve children. If one of the children became disturbed or aggressive, he – they were all boys – would be taken out off the ward, to appear later in the day much calmer.

There were also occasions when I had auditory hallucinations. These were not as dramatic as the visual ones I had had before I was admitted to St Lawrence's – the snapping mouths with sharp teeth – but were voices shouting at me. I would become very upset, and begin to beat my head against the floor. When I did this, two nurses would grab me and take me off the ward. My dressing gown and slippers were taken from me and I received an injection to calm me down. I was then placed in what the nurses called the 'quiet room'. This was a small room located in the corridor outside the ward. Ten feet by ten, it had no furnishings at all except a rubber mat that covered the floor. There was no window, no view, except for a small pane of glass in the door, at which a face regularly appeared to check on me. Being sedated meant I was usually doing nothing except sitting on the mat.

I – indeed every boy on my ward – was frightened of the quiet room, and by the middle of my time at St Lawrence's – that time when I was still ill enough, or became agitated enough, to be placed in the quiet room – I greatly feared it.

The quiet room was a nurse's warning: 'If you don't sit down Alex I'll put you in the quiet room'. 'If you don't calm down Alex we'll have to put you in the quiet room …' It was a threat that worked.

After about six weeks at St Lawrence's, every Saturday afternoon my father began to come to visit me, and I was taken downstairs to see him in a visitors' room. At the start of these meetings I was still very ill, and on the first occasions I became frantic, crying and pleading to be taken home, and usually ended up back in the quiet room for the rest of the afternoon.

It was very much a 'carrot and stick' method of mental care. If I remained calm and was no trouble, I was allowed to play with the collection of toys. If I misbehaved or became disturbed, which often extended to banging my head in frustration, then I was stripped of my dressing gown, and placed in the quiet room for several hours.

As the spring wore on to early summer, and my mental state was slowly restored, my life at St Lawrence's improved. Dr Smith instructed the nurses to stop putting me into my all-in-ones, and I was given pyjamas to wear. From about this time my father's visits every Saturday became the highlight of my week. He always came laden with bars of chocolate and went out of his way to cheer me up. This was a new experience for me, to be the focus of my father's attention without my mother's interference, and I think that these visits were incredibly important for both of us. In my case it was because I was able to develop a relationship with my father without my mother coming between us. For him,

I think he realised for the first time that if I could banish the mental illness I could be quite an interesting child.

Years later, as an adult, my father was to tell me that he had not really had enough input into my life by the time of my admission to St Lawrence's in 1973. It was only after he had started to see me for a few hours every Saturday that he saw that my mother was a malign influence on the family.

However, by the summer of 1973 my father had still not recognised how dangerous or treacherous my mother could be. He was still in love with a woman who was prepared to do anything to get her own way. It was not that my father was a weak man, he was just mild-mannered and still inclined to let her have her own way. This would continue until it was almost too late, not only for me, but him too.

CHAPTER 6

Athens

While I was slowly recovering in St Lawrence's Hospital events were beginning to take place in the Middle East in the summer of 1973 that would, indirectly, threaten my state of mind and lead to one of the most terrifying periods of my life. Western Intelligence evaluated that Egypt and Syria intended to attack Israel to seize back the Sinai Desert and Golan Heights lost to Israel in the 1967 Middle Eastern War. As a result the Foreign Office asked my father to act as an adviser at a military establishment near Cologne in West Germany, with special remit to liaise with the German government. My father accepted the appointment.

When my father returned from a meeting at the Foreign Office in London in August to announce he had accepted the post in West Germany on the basis of a one-year appointment, starting in September, my mother went berserk, accusing my father of abandoning her and the children; she screamed, she shouted, she threw things about the house. Vicky and I hid in Vicky's bedroom, and listened in fear to Mother's screamed obscenities, her declarations of betrayal echoing down the corridor.

By the time my father made this announcement, I was back at home. Having made good progress by June at St Lawrence's, I had been discharged on 15 July. After five months in hospital my homecoming was an anti-climax. Vicky hugged me, my father smiled a lot, but my mother could hardly bring herself to talk to me, let alone touch me. She shrank back when I went to her, and merely said 'hello', as if I had only been gone an hour.

Now, in August, I could see for myself the terrible arguments my parents had over my father's appointment in West Germany. However, despite my mother's violent rages, for once my father would not give in. His appointment in West Germany came with an Army house at the base. He tried to placate my mother by telling her that we all, as a family, could go to live in West Germany. My mother not only spurned his offer of family unity in Germany, she also refused to stay in Britain as well. She threatened to divorce my father if he went to Germany, but for once he called her bluff and would not give in.

Their arguments lasted days, until, in the end, my father finally relented. My mother insisted she wanted to take us children to live with Auntie Elle in Athens. After all, the rest of my mother's inheritance was still in Greece, and so my father reluctantly agreed to take us all to live with Auntie Elle for the duration of his appointment in West Germany. As a family, my mother, sisters, and I, were going to live in Athens for a year.

My life at home in August 1973 was much better than it had been before I'd been taken ill. I had been sent home from St Lawrence's with six pairs of padded cotton incontinence pants, much more comfortable than what my mother had made me wear, and was, in fact, having very few accidents by the time of my discharge.

Also, I was now, at the age of ten, allowed to wear normal pyjamas at home, not the awful anti-strip all-in-ones; nor was I locked in my room at night. I don't know what had been decided by my parents while I was in St Lawrence's, but I got the distinct impression that my father had told my mother to ease up on me. Could she have even blamed herself for my illness? Had my mental breakdown been worse than she had anticipated? I guess I'll never know, but once back home she very carefully gave me the correct doses of Chlorpromazine and Valium.

There was another situation that surprised me. On my return home in July I was astonished to discover that Vicky was now taller than me – and by quite a bit, too. To find that Vicky, at nine, was now taller than me aged ten, coupled with the fact that I was still sent to bed at 7.30 p.m. while she was allowed to stay up much later, made me very jealous.

Vicky now began to side with my mother against me. My mother had brainwashed her into believing that I was 'mental' and 'autistic', and she would fling these words at me, as well as other hurtful taunts, whenever my father was out of earshot. It now felt very much that the family was divided: my mother and sister on one side, my father and

I on the other. And soon, I was to be separated from my one ally.

On 3 September 1973, we set off on the 2,800-mile journey across Europe to Athens. Naturally I was very excited at the prospect of a foreign trip, never having been away from home in the motorhome. However, the pleasure was taken off the occasion for me because my clothing through the long journey was a canary-yellow nylon shirt and stretchy red jumpsuit, which I found very humiliating and hated.

Despite my not having to wear the hated all-in-ones any more, Dr Smith had told the nurses at St Lawrence's to continue the practice of making me wear my jumpsuits in the day, just in case the disordered thought occurred to me to strip, a habit sometimes seen in autistic children. My father had agreed to Dr Smith's instructions on my discharge, especially at my mother's insistence once I was home. He just didn't seem to be able to stand up to my mother where I was concerned, especially when she was backed up by my psychiatrist.

The journey across Europe took five days. There was a heat wave in Eastern Europe that year, and by the time we reached Yugoslavia the temperature was a terrific 38°C.

I was melting in my jumpsuit and nylon shirt, so my mother relented under my father's insistence, and took the jumpsuit off me. However, Chlorpromazine has a severe side effect: it makes one extremely light-sensitive and my skin erupted into hundreds of tiny blisters in strong sunlight. This meant that, despite the oppressive heat, I had to remain in my shirt and cover my bare legs with a towel.

Six days after setting out from home we arrived at my Aunt Elle's house in Athens on Sunday afternoon, the heat stifling at 40°C. The house seemed bigger than I remembered, a sprawling range of corridors and dim cool rooms, the pale-blue metal shutters pulled shut to keep out the worst heat of the day.

My aunts and uncles had not changed at all, but their five children all looked a lot older. The eldest, Eftihia, was now fourteen and towered over me; her brother, Theo, was a very tall twelve-year-old. The rest of my cousins, Spiros, Elizabeth, and Vasiliki, all aged between nine and eleven, were also taller than me.

Everyone was in their Sunday best clothes – white shirts for the boys, girls in white dresses. My uncles and father wore freshly laundered white shirts; my mother and aunts in light cool dresses. Virtually without exception everyone was dressed in white. Everyone that is, except me. I stood out like a brightly coloured stick of rock in my yellow shirt and red jumpsuit, feeling as embarrassed and incongruous as a circus clown among choristers.

I can remember thinking, 'I hate this. I don't want to stay here. I want to go to Germany with Dad!'

I didn't dare voice my thoughts.

We all flooded down the wide hall to the back of the house to spill out into the main big drawing room, where there were *metzethes* (olives, whitebait, and snacks) all laid out. The adults drank glasses of wine, we children glasses of lemonade.

Mother pushed me into a chair, and told me to stay

seated there, out of the sun that would blister my skin. Vicky vanished into the garden with our cousins, who seemed to want to have nothing to do with me. I found myself hoping this was not going to remain the case throughout our year-long stay, otherwise I was going to be very lonely.

After a short time, while the women chattered, my father and uncles went out to the Bedford to bring in the luggage. When my father and uncles came back more wine was poured, and they sat talking with much laughter.

It was at this time that my mother and Aunt Sophia – a pleasant woman in her thirties with long dark hair in a ponytail – left to take Ingrid for a bath. As a family we had not had a proper wash – except strip-washes – for nearly a week. Next Vicky was called in, and she too was taken off upstairs for a bath. After twenty minutes Vicky reappeared, refreshed. My mother now called me to come, and I found myself taken up the stairs to the top floor, which was where we would be staying.

It was after my bath that the first inkling that my life in Greece was going to swiftly become a living nightmare came to me. Dragged back to the bedroom with a towel around my waist, I found myself left standing while Mother rummaged in one of the suitcases on the floor.

To my anguish she now produced one of my large pads and a pair of the rubber pants. She snatched the towel away from me and told me to stand still. I was horrified as the pad and rubbers were roughly pulled on to me.

I stood there looking at my clothes, the shirt and jumpsuit lying on the bed, and waited for her to let me dress. Instead she returned to the suitcase and began to unpack it. To my absolute horror she now produced one of my pale-green all-in-ones.

'Here we are,' she said, grinning evilly at me. 'You'll wear these from now on.'

I instantly broke down. Sobbing, I pleaded with her not to make me wear the all-in-one, not in front of everyone, not in front of my aunts and uncles, and especially my cousins.

My mother took no notice and, with a savage expression on her face, pushed me on to the bed. After a brief struggle, she forced me into the long-johns, shoving my arms roughly down the sleeves. For once I really did struggle against her, flailing about, screaming and sobbing.

'Please,' I pleaded. 'Don't do this. Please, please, please, don't do this. I'm sorry, please don't!'

She shouted at me to be quiet, dragged me face down on the bed, and knelt on me while she struggled to do the large tight-fitting rubber buttons up the back.

When she eventually got off me, I just sat on the bed and sobbed. Suddenly I realised that her seeming compassion to me since I had come home from St Lawrence's – being allowed to wear pyjamas, using cotton inconto-pants – had all been a fraud, her scheme to deceive my father about how she intended to treat me from now on.

'I hate you,' she shrieked. 'I hate you, HATE you, you little *bastard*!'

I was shocked into silence. She'd often called me hurtful

and demeaning names in the past, but she'd never called me a 'bastard' before.

Grabbing my hair in both her hands as I struggled, she pulled me off the bed on to the floor and proceeded to beat me about the head and face. I was then left sobbing on the floor while she, as if nothing had happened, proceeded to tidy the room.

Eventually my mother finished what she was doing, and turned to me with that sinister smile she possessed playing on her lips. It wasn't a normal smile, more like a grimace, and it was at times like this I believe she was really very dangerous. She certainly terrified me.

Without a word, she pulled me up off the floor and, holding me in front of her by the scruff of the neck, pushed me from the room, across the landing, and down the stairs. I was nearly physically sick there and then in anxiety and fear of my mother, and because of the knowledge of the embarrassment and humiliation to come.

Arriving at the drawing room my mother gave me a hard shove into the room.

The conversation died and there was dead silence, as I stood there barefoot in my close-fitting all-in-one over the top of a very evident large pad.

My mother's laughter rang out, as jarring and foul as an obscenity shouted in church. I don't know what she expected to happen; don't know what she thought her relatives would say.

A lone voice broke the silence. It was my father's.

'Oh, Voula. For God's sake …'

He got no further, for my mother shrieked at him, 'Shut up! Shut up! *Shut up!*'

My father tried to interrupt, getting up and crossing the room to her.

'He's mental! He's retarded!' she shouted. 'He wets himself! You know he does. He's going to stay in a nappy now, and I won't have him stripping.'

She grabbed me, dragged me across the room, and forced me to sit on the floor next to an armchair.

'Don't you dare get up!' she warned me.

Tearfully, I looked over at the French doors, where my cousins and Vicky now stood gaping at the spectacle that was taking place.

'Voula,' my father interrupted. 'I want to talk to you …'

'Okay!' my mother snapped in a scream of anger.

She led the way out into the garden, and within moments came the sound of raised voices, my mother's shrieking off the scale. My father eventually lost his temper and the shouting became even more intense.

Auntie Elle ushered my cousins and Vicky through the room out to play elsewhere. I just sat on the floor, humiliated in front of everyone, and listened to my parents screaming at each other in the garden.

After ten minutes my mother returned, with a grim expression on her face. My father did not come back. He took himself for a long walk to escape the embarrassing situation and to calm down.

With my cousins and Vicky gone to play elsewhere, my mother became the centre of attention. She spoke at length to my aunts and uncles in Greek, pointing wildly at me occasionally, and there was much venom on her face. My aunts and uncles kept turning to stare at me, and no one was smiling any more. I think that my mother was effectively turning them against me, telling them I was mentally ill, autistic, and psychotic, that I wet myself, that I had been in a mental hospital all spring. Fear of the mentally ill was extremely prevalent in Greece at the time, and I could tell by the expressions on my aunts' and uncles' faces that they would support my mother, whatever she did to me.

My father was in an impossible situation. He had agreed to bring my mother and us children to Greece for the duration of his appointment in Germany. In the immediate aftermath of my discharge from St Lawrence's my mother had seemingly been reasonable towards me.

Had it all been a deceitful trick? Had she planned this all along?

All I knew was that I was terrified of my mother, and now with all her relatives looking askance at me I just wanted to leave there with my father and never come back.

Originally my father was to stay a few days in Athens, before his long lone journey across Europe to Britain, before packing what he needed to take to Germany. All that ended now. Things between him and my mother were so bad that he left the morning after the fight. In the front hall he gave Vicky a hug, and kissed Ingrid's head as my mother held her.

Finally he turned to me as I stood there barefoot in my all-in-one. His voice broke as he said goodbye to me, and he hugged me and hugged me. I thought he'd never let go.

Suddenly he was gone. He turned and went through the door, walking fast down the driveway. He did not look back; I think the emotion of the situation was too much for him. We did not go out to see him leave. All we saw was the roof of the Bedford in the road behind a high hedge, and then he was gone.

My mother slammed the door shut with a loud bang, then, talking to Vicky and carrying Ingrid, walked slowly back down the hall. I just stood there, feeling alone and very abandoned.

I had, the first night at Auntie Elle's house, slept in a twin room with Vicky. Now, the day Father left, my mother and her relatives showed me how they considered a mentally ill child, which is what I think they believed me to be, should be handled.

Uncle Stamatis, a clean-shaven man with long sideburns, dismantled my bed and put a cot in its place; Vicky was going to share her room with Ingrid. Next he cleared the small room across the second-floor landing from my mother's room until it was completely empty. He then placed my metal-framed bed in the room, the only other furniture a small bedside cupboard.

I watched as my mother supervised Uncle Stamatis's work in my room. The window, which was kept open because of the oppressive heat, had metal shutters with thin slats to let in some light. Stamatis drilled a hole in the shutters' latch, and secured it shut with a screw. They could not now be opened. Next he drilled a hole into the door-frame and affixed a stout bolt to the outside of the door. My mother, having informed her relatives that I was mad and unstable, had arranged that I could be locked securely in my room at night. Even the shutters were locked shut now, so that I wouldn't fall – or jump – out of the window. The room would always be dim from now on.

Just as when we had visited a few years earlier, and because there were now so many people living in the house – six adults and eight children – everyone was fed in order of age. We children had our meal at six o'clock; the adults of the house ate much later, at about eight.

Now, at 6 p.m. on Monday, the first full day at Auntie Elle's, all us children were summoned to the dining room for the main meal of the day. When I entered my mother grabbed my arm and shoved me into a chair.

The meal was brought in: a large dish of moussaka, which was plated out for us children. Eftihia, Vicky and the others were all given their meals, but my mother took my portion away to the kitchen. When she returned with my meal it was now slopped into a bowl and cut up into small pieces. My mother banged the dish down in front of me, snatched my knife and fork away, and handed me a spoon to use. My cousins looked at me in astonishment. Evidently I was so mental I was not capable of using a knife and fork.

I can remember I sobbed off and on through the entire meal that first evening. My cousins just stared at me as they ate, leaving the table to go and play as soon as they finished.

I just sat there, the last one at the table, until my mother eventually grabbed the spoon off me and crammed the last of the food into my mouth.

Once my meal was finished, even before she put Ingrid to bed, my mother hauled me away upstairs. After having my face rubbed over with a wet flannel, Mother made me take a handful of pills, many of them the anti-psychotic tranquilliser Chlorpromazine, and locked me in my room.

I spent hours that first evening standing at the window in the dying light, resting my head against the metal shutters and peering down through the narrow slits into the yard at the side of the house where Vicky and my cousins played with a ball. I sobbed for hours as I stood there, feeling very lonely indeed. Eventually I slumped on top of the bed and fell asleep.

That September in Athens I was treated by everyone as severely mentally impaired. Vicky was enrolled at the local school. She now spent all her time with my cousins and hardly gave me a second thought. She was even beginning to speak Greek, which she picked up very quickly. This left me all the more isolated because my mother insisted on speaking Greek to Vicky all the time, and I had no idea what anyone was talking about.

From the very first day I was left barefoot, dressed in a pad, rubbers, and all-in-one, twenty-four hours a day, seven days a week. Every day for the rest of that autumn and into the winter, my regime was exactly the same. Every morning I was left locked in my room until Vicky and my cousins left for school. My mother would then let me out, take me to the toilet, before doing the all-in-one securely up at the back. I was then taken down to the dining room where, sitting by myself, I had a bowl of porridge. I had to stay seated at the table until my mother came back, even if I was left there all morning.

My days were very repetitive. The men of the house worked, the children went to school at 8 a.m., and so, left with just the four women and Ingrid, I was told I had to stay in the sitting room – a smaller room with easy chairs, sofa, dining table, and TV – and play with toys on the floor. I used to sometimes wander the house, but every time I was spotted my mother and aunts would slap my legs and take me back to the sitting room. There was one rule among all the others made for me: under no circumstances was I allowed to step out of the house, not even for a moment.

By the afternoon, the Greek school day having ended at 2 p.m., my cousins and Vicky came home, and we had our lunch in the dining room. Vicky and my cousins would then go out to play all afternoon.

At 6 p.m. we children were gathered in the dining room for dinner. They were nice children, but gave me curious looks as I sat there in an all-in-one, eating my meal with a spoon. Once I finished my mother immediately pulled me from the table, and dragged me away to my room, where she forced me to take a large number of tablets. I soon didn't know what these tablets were, for my mother acquired them in Greece, so they could have been generic Chlorpromazine or Valium. They were certainly sedatives of some kind because they made me sleepy, and that was the end of my day.

I was now – it happened immediately my father left – forbidden to go anywhere near Ingrid. One day I was forcefully sat down, with all my aunts and uncles standing intimidatingly over me, and told I was not allowed to touch Ingrid, I was not to go near Ingrid, and I was not to play with Ingrid. My mother told me these things in English (a rarity), then spoke at length in Greek, translating her instructions to my aunts and uncles. This situation was to result in horrific repercussions for me, which occurred towards the end of September.

It was my mother's habit – Ingrid now being about eight months old and very active – to lay her on a quilt on the drawing-room floor for an hour most mornings. On this particular day I had been playing in the sitting room, but had got bored. I wandered down the long dark hall to the drawing room, intending to look out of the French doors at the rear garden. When I entered the drawing room I saw Ingrid lying on the quilt, happily waving her little arms and legs in the air. I went over to watch her. It didn't seem to do any harm so I sat next to her on the quilt and let her grab my finger with her tiny podgy hand. She made a happy little sound, and I just sat there gazing at her.

Suddenly there was a scream of anguish and, startled, I jumped up, snatching my hand away. I turned to see my mother standing in the doorway. She was furious, and ran across the room. The sudden noise of her outburst, or the act of me snatching my hand away, upset Ingrid and she started to cry.

My mother, quite hysterical by now, started screaming for help. She pounced on me and wrestled me flat on the floor.

Everything now seemed to happen in double time. My aunts came running, Auntie Elle picked Ingrid up off the quilt and took her to the corner of the room, where she sat rocking her. My mother was screaming frantically as if I'd tried to hurt or even murder Ingrid, and Auntie Sophia joined my mother in pinning me down. Terrified, I sobbed and struggled as the two adults held me face down on the floor. My mother shouted something in Greek. Auntie Kristina rushed away and returned with a pair of tights, which she and my mother used to bind my hands very tightly behind me. I struggled and screamed as I lay face down on the floor, but I could not fight off three adults. In the end my hands were bound, and my two aunts held me down while my mother rushed away to Ingrid. I watched sobbing as she ran her hands over my sister, stroking her head, and checking her fingers.

Satisfied Ingrid was okay, she came back over and, with my aunts, hauled me to my feet. She grabbed me from my aunts and shook and shook me, screaming in Greek at me. I was terrified.

With my aunts' help she dragged me away up the stairs to my room. There my mother forced me to take a handful of tablets. Then my aunts pinned me face down on my bed, and held me there while my mother left the room. There was much shouting – again in Greek – between my mother and aunts, before she returned clutching several pairs of tights and a belt. As I lay sobbing, the tights were looped through my arms at the elbow, and then pulled very tight and tied to the metal frame of the bed at the sides, so I could not move or turn over. Next my ankles were strapped together with the belt, and then secured to the bars at the foot of the bed. They let go of me, snatching the pillow away, and stood watching as I struggled on the bed. I screamed and cried, but they just left me there, closing the door behind them. I sobbed and screamed for what seemed an eternity until, the pills finally taking effect, I subsided into silence.

I must have spent the whole day tied to my bed and had fallen asleep like that, for when I eventually woke up, my mother and Uncle George were in my room untying me.

Between the two of them they got me off the bed and to my feet, but I was very uncoordinated, as I was taken from my room and downstairs. As we got downstairs to the hall, I saw myself in the large wall mirror, and was shocked. My hair was standing on end, and I looked very pale and small between my mother and George.

Taken into the dining room, my bare feet stumbling on the floor, I was pushed on to a chair. Vicky and my cousins were just finishing their meal. A spoon was placed in my hand, and my mother stood over me as I attempted to feed myself. I was groggy, still sedated, and my hands so numb and uncoordinated that I was getting in a real mess. My mother snatched the spoon from my hand, loaded it up, and crammed it into my mouth. I gagged and half the food fell out, but she persisted until it was all gone.

As soon as the meal was finished, I was dragged back upstairs, where I was stripped. Stood over by my mother and George, I was made to use the toilet and then changed. I was put back into the same food-splattered, stale all-in-one, given a second large number of tablets, then locked back in my room.

Despite the fact that my mother had brought several all-in-ones with her – and virtually no other clothes – for me to wear, she only gave me a clean one to wear once a fortnight, sometimes even less often. I was always unclean, stale and sweaty. I'm sure this was done to humiliate and degrade me; there seemed no practical purpose it could serve. I had failed my mental assessments, and due to the psychological stress and drug abuse she had inflicted on me, I had suffered psychosis. Now I was kept unclean and smelly. My mother was determined to exact her own particular type of insane revenge on me for not being perfect, like Vicky – a pliant living doll. She just did not seem to accept me as a boy; from my earliest days she had been hard on me. This was especially so since I failed my mental assessments. Perhaps she had not wanted a son. Perhaps in her unstable mind she related me to her brother, Yiannis, who *was* mentally handicapped, and had been rejected and effectively thrown away by her parents. I was never to learn the answer to why she hated me so much, but I'm sure it lies somewhere between all of these possibilities.

Once a week an elderly Greek Orthodox priest, in long black robes and a beard, visited my aunts and mother. On the first occasion I met him, I remember I was stale and unclean. Despite his religious calling he looked at me, dressed in a nappy underneath a dirty food-splattered all-in-one, with something like disgust on his face. Although I spoke no Greek, I could tell from my mother's voice that I was once again labelled as the mental child; unfit to be educated, kept at home and tolerated by my pious relatives. The elderly priest put his hand on my head and muttered some religious incantation, then crossed himself.

Ever since that first meeting I was kept out of the way whenever the priest came to visit, put in the sitting room while he sat in the drawing room with my aunts and mother, drinking strong black coffee and talking earnestly about religion. Very occasionally it happened that I'd meet him in the hall as he left. If I stood hesitantly before the priest, half prepared to plead for help, I was grabbed by Mother or my aunts, and bundled into the sitting room, the door slammed shut behind me.

I was acutely aware I was alone and isolated in a country thousands of miles from my father with people who treated me with contempt.

After my father left Athens in early September, he had driven back across Europe to Britain on his own. On reaching home he had loaded up the Bedford with his books, papers, and clothes, then set off to drive to West Germany, arriving at the military establishment near Cologne in mid-September.

My father had been there only a week when he received

a letter from my mother. In a brief note she declared that she was not going to return to Britain, and demanded a divorce. All future correspondence would be through her lawyer.

Devastated, my father now realised he had been tricked by my mother; deviously she had planned this all along. My father knew the Greek authorities were tough when it came to Greek citizens and their children. They never gave custody of children to foreign nationals, and my father realised there was a chance he might never see my sisters or me again.

I had been in Athens about a month, it now being the middle of October, when yet another terrifying situation began to develop for me.

Every Saturday the whole family – mother, sisters, uncles, aunts, and cousins – went out for the entire day. They would leave in a convoy of cars around mid-morning to visit relatives for lunch and stayed out until the evening. As I was considered mentally deranged and not allowed out of the house, my mother, aunts, and uncles took turns to stay at home to look after me.

The aunt or uncle delegated to stay at home with me completely ignored me. Occasionally I'd be made to sit with them to watch the television, but since I didn't understand anything that was said, I had no interest in what was happening onscreen.

This was a very abnormal – and isolating – environment for me.

Many years later, as an adult, my psychiatrist would explain to me that this situation where I could not understand what was said, could not read books, and didn't even understand anything on television, was an artificially isolating and impairing 'autistic-type' environment. This was especially important when he considered that, as a consequence of my mother's abuse, I had developed a propensity to psychosis and withdrawal into my own closed-in world, things that were often diagnosed in those days as 'autistic traits'.

As time was to go on and I was badly treated for months, not spoken to, treated as mentally impaired, virtually unable to communicate, sedated and locked away in my room at the slightest disturbance, I began to get more and more unstable. I suffered severe episodes when I would flop on the floor sobbing, and beat my head against walls and doors. All this added together to present me as a mentally disturbed child.

Whenever I suffered one of these episodes, my aunts, uncles, and mother would pile in and pin me down on the floor. My hands were tightly bound behind me and I'd be dragged away screaming to my room, where I'd be sedated and tied face down on my bed, bound at elbows and ankles, for the rest of the day. I would scream hysterically at the top of my lungs, but no one ever came back until the evening, or sometimes even the next day.

My Auntie Elle's eldest son, Uncle Manolis, an officer in the merchant navy, came home for a few days once a fortnight. I remembered him from our first visit to Athens, how impressive he was in his uniform.

In November Uncle Manolis began to stay at home with me every other Saturday. I liked Uncle Manolis because he was the only adult who did not treat me badly. He would always come home in his smart officer's uniform, cap and jacket with gold braid, and I liked him.

However, at home Manolis always stripped off his uniform and sat around in a T-shirt drinking bottles of beer.

I suppose I was a very naïve child because what happened next I misconstrued as kindness, starved as I was of affection.

On the first Saturday Manolis stayed home with me, he made me sit on the sofa next to him in the sitting room during the afternoon. There was some incomprehensible film on the television, so I quickly lost interest.

On the next Saturday Manolis and I were alone, he held me tight and talked to me. Then, to my surprise, he undid the buttons down the back of my all-in-one, and took it off me. I sat next to him on the sofa while he put his arm around me. I can remember my embarrassment at wearing rubber pants and a pad in front of him. This situation now began to occur every other Saturday; he would let me out of my all-in-one for a few hours, but was always careful to re-dress me before my mother returned.

This was our big secret, and I – a very lonely and innocent child – began to look forward to our times together. The only thing I didn't like was that he began to make me sit on his lap. Even I knew that this was inappropriate for a ten-year-old boy. However, I did not in my naïve way realise exactly what was happening. I was just glad someone was giving me some attention and being nice to me for a change.

Christmas of 1973 came, and I watched in envy as my cousins and Vicky laughed and chattered away in high-speed Greek as they decorated the large Christmas tree in the drawing room and put up decorations around the house.

I felt really strange a lot of the time now. I don't think I was mentally at all well. Occasionally I would hear a 'voice' talking to me, and sometimes it came out of the television, which meant that I was once again suffering from auditory hallucinations. I also increasingly became frantic and beat my head against walls or floor. Even though my mental state was clearly getting worse, I never saw a doctor the whole time I lived at my Auntie Elle's. I could not understand anything that was said to me, my mother was harsh with me, and I was increasingly very confused a lot of the time.

Christmas morning came, and my mother borrowed my cousin Spiros's dressing gown and put it on me to hide my stale all-in-one while she photographed Vicky, Ingrid, and me opening our presents; the idea being to send the pictures to my father in West Germany. The dressing gown was immediately taken off me as soon as I had been photo-graphed.

I had my Christmas lunch seated by myself in the sitting room. I was ignored all afternoon while a great buffet was laid out in the dining room. I played with my new toys and watched a cartoon on the television, all by myself. In the late afternoon my mother came in with a meal for me, which I again had by myself seated at the table. Directly after finishing my meal I was taken away upstairs and made ready for bed. It was only 5 p.m., but that was the end of my Christmas Day. There was to be a big party that evening, but I was not to attend as I was an embarrassment. Given a lot of tablets to keep me quiet, I was put in my room, the door firmly locked by my mother as she left.

On the following morning no one came to let me out of my room. Everyone overslept because of the previous evening's celebration, which had lasted late into the night. After what seemed like many hours my mother eventually came to let me out, but instead of letting me use the toilet, I was hurriedly bundled down the stairs directly to the dining room, and made to sit with Vicky and my cousins who were already gathered for lunch. They were all smartly dressed for Christmas; I was in a grubby all-in-one I had worn for a month. I had become a stale and unclean mental child, and no one wanted me around.

Later that afternoon I was again made to sit and eat my tea by myself at the table in the sitting room, supervised by Eftihia, who had been told to make sure I didn't get up. Immediately I finished my meal my mother took me upstairs and locked me in my room, out of sight and out of mind. There was another big party that evening, and I could hear laughter and music wafting up through the house to the top floor. I had a good weep, wondering about my father. Was he at a party that Boxing Day evening? Would he ever come to take me home?

Christmas soon passed, and with the arrival of January my sister and cousins returned to school, my uncles returned to work, and I was again left at home with my mother and aunts.

My mental state had severely deteriorated by now. My bursts of emotional distress when I would frantically beat my head against the walls or floor became more and more frequent. None of this did me any good, nor did it present me in a good light to my mother, aunts, or uncles.

Several weeks after Christmas a Saturday came when I was again left in the care of Uncle Manolis. I had by now begun to be wary of my uncle, for although I did not mind him taking my all-in-one off me for a few hours, the fact that he made me sit on his lap in just my rubber pants sent an alarm bell ringing in my mind.

It had snowed heavily that weekend in Athens. Because it was chilly in the house I was not keen on sitting unclothed on my uncle's lap. I suppose I had become resigned to my fate. Every adult I knew did just what they wanted to me: from treating me as mentally handicapped and disordered all the time, sedating and restraining me if I became frantic or disturbed, to Uncle Manolis taking my clothes off me and 'fingering' me as I sat on his lap.

Everyone had left for their Saturday trip out, and I found myself alone with Uncle Manolis. Initially he went outside into the snow, and I watched him from the window as he fiddled with his car, which was parked in the yard at the side of the house.

After a long time Manolis came in and made some lunch,

which we had seated at the table in the kitchen. Directly after lunch we went into the sitting room, where he put the television on. There was a war film on, babbled in Greek I didn't understand, nor had any interest in, so I took myself off into the corner to play.

It was at this point that Manolis called me over. He made me stand before him as he sat on the sofa and, turning me around, undid the buttons of my all-in-one. It dropped down around my ankles, and I expected to be pulled to sit on his lap as usual.

Instead, to my surprise, before I realised what he was doing, Manolis dropped my rubbers and pad down around my ankles, and I stood naked before him. I was used to being naked in front of my mother and aunts, but never before in front of Manolis.

He made me sit on his lap while he continued to watch the television. This all seemed to last a long time, and by now I was very perturbed indeed by the way he held me. I had a sick feeling deep in the pit of my stomach, and was shaking nervously.

Suddenly, to my surprise, Manolis stood up and picked me up off the floor. He was a very strong man, and carried me effortlessly across the room to the table.

I was very frightened by now. He placed me face down on the table. I struggled briefly, but my feet did not reach the floor. Next he draped himself over me. He was very heavy, smelt of cigarettes, and, terrified, I began to cry out. A large hand was firmly placed over my mouth and he pinched my nose shut with his thumb and forefinger. I sobbed silently, struggling to breathe, squirming under him and trying to get away. But he was too strong and heavy, and I was effectively trapped.

I could feel him doing something to my backside, and suddenly I was in terrific pain. I wanted to cry out, but could not force the air out of my lungs and mouth.

The pain became excruciating and I gave a muffled scream.

Suddenly there was the noise of a door slamming in the house, the sound of voices. In an instant Manolis was off me and across the room. Sobbing in fear, I could not comprehend what had happened, and I slid off the table to stand trembling on the floor.

At that moment my mother entered the room, and Manolis began shouting angrily at her, and pointing wildly at me standing naked in the corner.

My mother too flew into a rage, and she began shouting at me as well. I did not know what I had done. I tried to tell my mother that Manolis had undressed me and he had hurt me. That my backside hurt very much …

I got no more than a few words out before she let out a tremendous scream, and slapped my face as hard as she could, knocking me to the floor. Extremely shocked, I knelt gasping in pain on the floor.

She grabbed a handful of my hair, dragging me across the floor, and slapping my backside as hard as she could in a frenzy.

I looked up to see my aunts, uncles, and cousins standing in the doorway, open-mouthed.

I'm sure Manolis was shouting something along the lines

of: 'Mad child! He's taken his clothes off!' and 'It's nothing to do with me!'

Still held by my hair, I was pulled to my feet and dragged naked and sobbing from the room past staring uncles, aunts, and cousins. Traumatised and crying in pain and fear, I was dragged upstairs to my room. Giving me a tremendous shove into my room and a hard slap across the head, my mother slammed the door shut behind me and locked me in. My head hurt where she'd pulled my hair, my face stung where I'd been slapped, and my backside felt as if it was on fire because of what Manolis had done to me. I broke down sobbing, terrified in case my mother came back and wondering what she was going to do to me.

It was at this point that I snapped. I looked wildly about the room. Spotting an empty glass on the bedside cabinet, I picked it up and threw it with all my strength against the wall, where it smashed with an explosive bang.

I was quite frantic by now, terrified about what my mother would do to me when she returned. My mother didn't care about me; she cared only for my sisters. I knew she hated me; she had told me enough times.

I picked up a large piece of broken glass, the heavy thick base that had a long sharp four-inch knife-like shard projecting out. Without a moment's hesitation, and in a quite demented way, I slashed the glass hard against my face and neck in one swift cutting blow. I didn't feel anything, and so I plunged the blade into the base of my abdomen. It went in up to the hilt. Again, I felt nothing. I pulled the glass out and dropped it on the floor.

It was at this moment that I noticed a great welling of blood pouring down my chest from the wound in my face and neck. There was also a lot of blood gushing from my abdomen that ran down my legs and dripped to pool on the floor. For the first time I felt a sensation like fire in my face and an agonising pain in my stomach.

I began to scream at the top of my lungs.

Suddenly the door flew open with a bang, and there stood my mother. The look of hatred on her face instantly turned to one of horror. She put her hands to her face and began to scream as well.

Within moments my aunts and uncles appeared at the door. My Uncle George took one look at me and rushed into the room, pushing past my hysterical mother. He snatched the blanket off my bed and wrapped it around me like a cocoon. He swept me off my feet, and carried me down the stairs. He was shouting instructions now, and he, together with my mother and Uncle Stamatis, rushed me from the house out to the car.

As I looked back over my uncle's shoulder, I saw my Auntie Elle in tears standing in the snow at the front door, my cousins gaping open-mouthed at what was happening. I was never to see them or that house ever again.

CHAPTER 7

Committed

Everything was white as I lay in bed staring around my room. White walls, white door, white cupboard, chair, and screen, even a white bedstead and bedding. The only splash of colour was me as I snuggled comfortably in bed in blue pyjamas.

This was the Agia Sophia Hospital, the main general hospital of Athens.

The day that Uncle Manolis assaulted me, following which, highly distressed and almost out of my mind, I had cut myself, my Uncles George and Stamatis and my mother had rushed me to the hospital. I don't remember much about the rest of that day. As soon as we arrived I was immediately sedated because I was completely hysterical and couldn't be calmed down.

I had been in hospital for two weeks, and I lay in bed, safe in the knowledge that I was surrounded by people who took care of me, and were nice to me. Every half hour a nurse opened my door to check I was okay, but I was not allowed to leave my room. At the beginning of my stay I was very disturbed, sobbing for hours on end, hiding in the corner and screaming every time anyone came near me. Now I was kept lightly sedated to minimise those times when I would kneel beside my bed and beat my head against the floor. When I did this the nurse would call for help, and I'd be picked up off the floor and held on the bed until I calmed down.

A large sticking plaster covered one cheek and extended down my neck. There was also a large plaster across my stomach. My face, neck, and abdomen had been sewn back together; seventy stitches in all. The stitches were out now, and I was on the way to physical recovery.

My mental state was not good, however. I was very agitated, tearful all the time, I had been abused by my uncle; without my father, my mother had waged a war on my body and mind for four long months and I was in a very poor state indeed. It didn't take much to disturb me, and when I was in such a state I would beat my head against the floor or a wall.

During that fortnight in the hospital I had only seen my mother twice. On the first occasion she came soon after my admission, but I became so distraught, refusing to let her near me and, screaming, backed into the corner of the room, that she gave up in disgust and stormed out.

When she came a week later, Uncle Manolis brought her, and there was a doctor present too. In terror of my mother and Manolis, thinking they had come to take me back to Auntie Elle's, I became hysterical, screaming at them to stay away, and actually hid under the bed sobbing. As I sobbed under the bed, my mother had a long conversation with the doctor. Eventually a decision was reached because they all started nodding and left.

With the passing days my conviction grew that my father would come for me. I had no firm foundations for this belief. Indeed, I was completely unaware my parents were in the process of divorce. I did not know that my father, far away in West Germany, had no idea about what was going on in Greece. If I had known these important details, perhaps I would have realised how precarious my situation was.

By now it had been a few days since my mother's last visit. It was a sunny morning in Athens, the sunlight streamed in through the window, illuminating my room in blinding whiteness. I lay curled up in bed, content just to sit and do nothing. It was then, at this time of relative peace and calm, that I was, without warning, taken from this safe place where I was cared for into a place that would shatter my life.

As I sat in bed, the door of my room was suddenly opened and two men were shown in by a nurse. What immediately struck me was that the two men were not smartly dressed like the doctors. Both wore open-necked shirts, one in a white jacket, the other in brown.

They stood talking for a moment as I sat staring at them, then brown-jacket opened the cupboard and pulled out the clothes my mother had brought. Without a word to me, the two men pulled me from the bed, took my pyjamas off me, and proceeded to dress me in trousers, jumper, and shoes. The men didn't bother with my shirt or socks, which they left discarded on the bed.

Then I was taken from my room, along the corridor, down the stairs, and out of the hospital. I was extremely anxious by now, fearing these men were taking me home to my mother. I had already worked out that white-jacket was no doctor, but I still did not know who these men were. I pulled back in the hospital foyer, on the edge of tears, and refused to go on, but I was unceremoniously hustled from the building.

The two men bundled me into the back of a red car, white-jacket sitting next to me and brown-jacket taking the wheel. Within seconds we were out of the hospital car park, and out in the traffic of a busy street. By now I was terrified that I was being taken home to my mother, and I began to weep. I rested my face against the glass and, sobbing, looked out at the world as it swept past.

We seemed to travel for a long time, the apartment blocks and shops becoming less numerous, until I realised we were leaving Athens. I was very worried by now. Perhaps these men have mistaken me for someone else? I thought as the car sped along, leaving Athens far behind. I had not the faintest idea where we were going, and my frantic attempts to talk to the men, to plead, sobbing, to be taken back, fell on deaf ears.

Eventually the car turned in through a big gateway. There was a sign outside, but not being able to read Greek I had no idea what it said. The car slowed down and drove through an extensive establishment of many big buildings, along narrow roads with high uncut grass at the side. The buildings all had an aura of dilapidation and neglect about them.

Although I did not know it then, nor indeed did I ever learn the name of this place during my whole time there, this was the Attica State Mental Institution, one of the largest mental hospitals in Greece. Greek mental healthcare has come on a long way since then and the present Attica Institution bears no resemblance to how it was then.

Built in 1920, the Attica Institution housed 2,000 men, women, and children, all considered to be chronic cases; a place the mentally disordered and handicapped were abandoned to the care of the State, and forgotten.

One day, long in the future, my father would tell me that he had learnt from my mother that when she had come with Manolis, she told the doctor – a psychiatrist – my mental history. She told him that I suffered psychosis, that I had been assessed in Britain as having severe mental disorder. On this basis – the autism, my psychosis, and the self-injury; she even showed the psychiatrist my Mental Health Certificate – he and my mother agreed that I should be committed. This was to be no short-term admission. The psychiatrist assessed my mental condition as severe and chronic, and my mother signed papers for my committal to the Attica State Mental Institution to be on a permanent basis: I could be here for the rest of my life.

Completely unaware of these facts, I was by now quite terrified of what was happening. The car stopped before a big building. I was pulled out and bundled in through a door. White-jacket and brown-jacket each grasped an arm, as I was taken through a locked metal gate, and down a long corridor. The whole place smelt unpleasant, like unclean public toilets.

After several corridors, white-jacket pushed open a door and I was taken into a tiled room. It was a big washroom with two dusty baths that had not been used in years. Brown-jacket left, while white-jacket proceeded to pull my clothes off me until I was standing naked and shivering before him. Brown-jacket reappeared carrying something that he dumped on the floor. I was pushed to sit on a stool and white-jacket produced a pair of clippers. Within a few minutes my mop of seventies-style hair was shorn off, and I was left with a crew-cut only a few millimetres long.

Brown-jacket picked the bundle up off the floor and let it fall open to reveal a tatty grey tieback cotton gown. It was pulled on to me and tied at the back of my neck. White-jacket grasped me firmly by my arm and led me – barefoot, sobbing, and cold, my backside open to the air – down long corridors, then up a flight of stairs to the first floor. The whole place was very dilapidated, with flaking cream paint on the walls, pale-blue paint on rails and doors, my feet padding along dirty floors, a mixture of concrete and well-worn tiles.

Eventually we stopped and white-jacket knocked on a blue door. Almost immediately it was opened by a woman wearing a pale-green wrap over her clothes. A few words were exchanged in Greek, then white-jacket handed me over to the woman, who pulled me into the room.

The first thing that hit me as I entered the room was the smell, an unpleasant mixture of disinfectant and excrement. The next thing that hit me – as if by delayed shock – was the sight that met my eyes. In the room were fifteen boys of about my age, some in tatty grey gowns like mine, several completely naked, some wandering aimlessly in the big room, others sitting on the floor rocking and making terrible noises. All this took just a few brief seconds for me to take in.

I heard the door shut behind me. I turned to see the woman lock the door and place the key in her pocket. I broke down crying, hysterically pulling at the door handle and trying to get out. The woman slapped me hard across my head and dragged me into the middle of the room where the severely mentally impaired children sat, and left me there. She returned to a seat by the door next to a second wrap-clad woman, and they began to gossip.

I had a good cry for several minutes, but while I stood there I had a chance to take in the sights of this awful place. None of the boys was clean, those clothed wore dirty gowns, those naked had excrement stains on their bodies and legs. All had their hair shorn off. The naked boys seated in the middle of the floor were the particularly sad cases. They rocked and made constant ululating noises; one was sitting in a pool of his own urine.

There was no care here. It was merely a place where mentally ill and handicapped children, some of whom had very severe problems, were accommodated. The women were not trained nurses, just locals hired to supervise the patients and to make sure that some sort of order was maintained.

Once I calmed down, I decided to explore my terrible new home.

The day room was very big, about 30 feet by 18 feet.

Walls once painted cream had faded and flaked. Along one wall, too high up to see out of, were windows set near the ceiling, well out of reach to be broken. It was the only source of natural light. At the far end of the room were two refectory tables with four benches.

By the locked door the two women sat on the only two chairs in the room, and behind them several belts hung on the wall. At this end of the room was the entrance to a corridor. I went into the corridor. On the left was a doorless entrance to a large washroom. There was a large stoneware sink to one side with a bucket, mops, and a few sodden rags hung to dry. On the other side of the room was a ceramic squat-toilet set into the floor, with a place on either side for your feet.

Back in the corridor, on the opposite side to the toilet room, were two doors, the lower half sheet steel and the upper half bars, painted once long ago pale blue. Both doors were padlocked shut.

I looked into the first room. It was a small room about ten feet square, there was no window, and it was dim and completely bare. In the corner squatted a naked child who rocked and kept hitting his head with his hands. I was to discover this boy was never let out. He stayed here the whole time I was in this place, fed there, left to go to the toilet in there, and only brought out every other day to be washed down with a wet rag. He never spoke, but made a lot of noise, especially at night, when he would yell and scream. He was completely insane, and I think he was permanently locked up because he was violent.

The second padlocked cell was identical to the first, but empty.

At the end of the corridor was an open door, so I ventured in. It was another large room, again dirty, dilapidated, and smelt like dirty public lavatories.

This room, again with the windows set near the ceiling, was full of adult-sized metal cots with high-lift sides. Each cot had a bare red rubber mattress and a screwed-up greasy-looking brown blanket. There was no other bedding and no pillows. I noticed that the majority of the cots had long strips of bandage tied to the four corners. The room was full of these cots in three rows, one down either side and a row in the middle, with not much space between them. The room was overcrowded.

Just as I turned to leave, I heard a noise from the far end, a child's voice crying out. I hadn't noticed him when I walked in. The boy lay naked upon the rubber mattress, his wrists and ankles tied tightly with the strips of bandage so he was spreadeagled on the cot. He turned his face to look at me, and I saw that he had one eye turned, giving him a boss-eyed look. I backed nervously away from him and he began to cry out, to scream and thrash violently about in his cot.

I fled the dormitory and ran back to the day room.

I spent the rest of the afternoon with my back against the wall, watching the children mill about. Several of them wandered back and forth like caged animals, and others squatted on their haunches rocking themselves. One of these, who was naked, would scream from time to time and beat his head with his hands.

The only children I did not fear were the six very mentally impaired boys sat on the floor in the middle of the room, who made constant ululating noises, as if the sound of their own voices comforted them. These boys were particularly pathetic cases. They were left naked because they kept soiling themselves, and thus received a lot of attention from the two women, who kept cleaning them up. It was doubtful if they knew where they were, and probably never would.

After what seemed like a very long time – during which I broke down sobbing several times – there was a bang on the door. The women roused themselves, and opened the door to admit a different white-jacketed man pushing a trolley with a big metal pot upon it. The women set to picking the very impaired boys up off the floor and sat them at the table, and slowly the other children followed. I was made to sit at the end of a bench next to a dirty naked boy who kept jumping and shrugging.

I was hungry by now, despite my distress, and I wondered what the meal was. Eventually a bowl and spoon were placed before me containing mashed food that may have been potato, swede, and carrots. It was lukewarm and bland, but there was nothing else, so I ate it.

I was never to discover during my whole time there what the food was. It was just mashed vegetables, or occasionally a thin stew. Drink was water handed out three times a day in plastic beakers.

Eventually, as each child finished, he left the table, to wander, squat, or sit about the corners of the day room. It took a long time for the two women to finish feeding the six very impaired boys, helping each one from the bench and placing him back on the floor in the middle of the room.

Bedtime in this place was early, just a short while after the evening meal. I had expected to be able to wash my face or swill my mouth out with water before bed, but these basic elements of hygiene were neglected here. Once in the dormitory I was directed to a cot, made to climb up on it; the side was raised, and that was it: I was left to my own devices. I looked at a child in the cot next to me, lying down, blanket covering him. Suddenly I realised his hands and feet had been bound to the cot with the strips of bandage. I immediately lay down and covered myself with the greasy blanket, determined that I should give no excuse to be tied to my cot.

After all the boys were placed in their cots the women left, closing the door behind them. I sobbed to myself long and hard that evening, cold, miserable, and feeling very alone.

When it eventually got dark I climbed out of my cot to try to escape. However, I discovered the dormitory door was locked. Some of the boys got very agitated when I walked past, screaming at me, so I hurried back to my cot and stayed there till morning. It was an unsettled night because some of the boys made terrible noises, calling out and shrieking. I could also hear a lot of distant noise from the lone boy in the cell, who became very disturbed indeed. He screamed and shouted all night.

I shivered most of that first night in the pitch dark; it was very chilly trying to sleep on a bare rubber mattress dressed only in a thin knee-length cotton gown and covered with a small blanket. However, the real reason I shook that night was fear. Fear that my mother had sent me here; fear that my father did not know what had happened to me. I prayed that night as I lay there that my father would come, and come soon, because I didn't know how much I would be able to take.

The daily routine in this place was very regimented.

The two women always came back to the dormitory some time after dawn. None of the boys ever got out of their cots until told to do so or, if tied down, released. The smell in the dormitory was bad by morning because some of the boys had wet and soiled themselves during the night. Those children were taken to the toilet room and washed down with a rag and cold water. The two women then engaged in their morning task of wiping off the soiled mattresses with a rag and bucket of cold water. Even I could tell it was not very hygienic.

We were left to ourselves in the day room, where virtually without exception the majority of boys returned to sitting or kneeling on the floor, rocking to comfort themselves in a small way. A few milled about all day, occasionally flapping their hands and becoming very agitated. One boy spent every day standing in the corner by himself facing the wall and rocking manically; he just soiled himself where he stood.

The exception to this general behaviour was a fragile-looking boy with big brown eyes and a solitary manner about him, who spent most of the day seated on his own on one of the benches. I soon discovered he was extremely epileptic, and had fits almost every day, sometimes even two or more, when he would collapse to the floor shaking. The two women would rush over and turn him into a particular position, and hold him still. There seemed to be something else wrong with him as well, because he could be very aggressive on some days, and would lash out if you went near him. In Greece prior to the 1980s it was not uncommon for epileptics to be placed in institutions, and I am sure his incarceration was detrimental to his mental well-being.

I soon found that there was no order to which cot I ended up placed in when it was time to sleep. In five days I was put to bed in five different cots. This was particularly unpleasant because I often ended up in a cot with an unclean smelly blanket, and the knowledge that this cot had probably been soiled the previous night and merely washed off with a rag and cold water was disgusting.

This was the regime in the Attica. It never varied from day to day. I never saw any other adults except for the two women who were there in the day, and the white-jacket who brought the meals. The two women never talked to the children in any way. They chattered between themselves, made sure everyone sat at the table for their meals, cleaned up if any child soiled himself, and at the end of the day put everyone to bed. That was the total extent of their interaction with us.

★

After about a week of being in this place, one morning the women went about the day room taking the gowns off everyone until we were all naked. Then, after a long while, three white-jackets arrived, and all us boys were herded out into the corridor. We were taken down the stairs, and then along a corridor until we came to a washroom. It was a big tiled room with two baths, and a big alcove behind a wall to one side that you had to step down a foot to get into.

Six boys were taken and pushed down into the alcove. One of the men turned a hosepipe on them, and they collectively let out an anguished cry and bent over or hugged the wall. The hosing stopped and the two women waded into the boys, armed with hand-brushes that they used to scrub at backsides, arms and legs; soap was something I never saw at the Attica. Then the hosepipe was again turned on them for a final rinse off.

After this, one boy at a time was grasped roughly by one of the men and taken over to a bath filled with pale-green water. He was made to kneel in the water, and then, grasped firmly by the back of the neck, pushed under the water and held there for several seconds. He emerged, screaming or sputtering, to be pulled out of the bath, and made to stand against the wall by the door.

When my turn came to be hosed down with a group of boys I found the water was freezing cold and I too cried out, bending over, and trying to get out of the way. I too had my backside painfully scrubbed with a stiff brush, and was hosed again.

Then a white-jacket grabbed me and I was dragged over to the bath, my wet feet slipping on the floor so that I almost fell. The pale-green water was not only freezing cold, but it smelt strongly of disinfectant. Plunged under for what seemed an eternity, I too emerged spluttering and screaming, because the disinfectant water stung agonisingly at my eyes and in my nostrils. I was then pulled out and shoved against the wall with the other boys, where a shivering queue gradually grew.

Eventually, this band of boys was herded naked, wet, and shivering, back along the corridors, up the stairs, and into the day room. Gowns were put back on some of the boys (half the boys were left naked all the time because they messed themselves so often), and I found myself wearing someone else's gown, which was dirty with another boy's faeces. Clean gowns were only handed out every second week, the same time as clean blankets were put upon the cots.

One day, after being in this terrible place nearly a month, I was kneeling on the floor in the corner of the day room when the epileptic boy came over and knelt next to me. He smiled and began to talk in Greek. I did not understand anything he said, but looking into his dark eyes and taking in the smile on his face, I realised he was trying to be friendly. He was an interesting and delicate-looking child, with an elfin pointed face and small aquiline nose.

I talked for the first time in weeks, told him in English that I did not understand what he said; I shook my head in the international gesture of non-comprehension.

The child looked blankly at me for a moment, then began to talk again, pointing at himself and repeating over and over again a single word: 'Nikki.'

I did the same, telling him my name, and he laughed. It was the first laugh I had heard in this dreadful place.

During the time I had spent here I had become very depressed. There was no respite from the routine of meals, bedtime, weekly washes, and interminable periods of boredom, broken only by having to endure the occasional outbursts of screaming by the demented children. One time I became desperate and shouted at the women that I wanted to go home. I was quite hysterical, screaming and sobbing at them, pounding my hands on the locked ward door. They just pushed me to sit on the floor in the middle of the room with the demented boys. Their verdict on me: mad child.

But now that I had made contact with Nikki I began to spend all my days with him, often sat on a bench at the table, not conversing, but just company for each other. Occasionally he would talk at length, but I didn't understand. In return I would tell him that I was sure my father was going to come for me. It was a way of assuring myself that someday I would get out of this asylum, and even though Nikki couldn't understand me, it comforted me to have someone to voice my hopes and fears to in this hopeless place. I would never know, but perhaps he was doing the same thing.

Once we spent the afternoon with him drawing pictures of a boat and fish with a spit-laden finger upon the table, repeatedly saying 'Babas.' I think that he was trying to tell me that his father was a fisherman. He then looked at me meaningfully, and pointed. I looked blank. What could I draw to show Nikki what my father did? It was not possible. Conversation died that afternoon, and we both sat silently together, alone with our own thoughts of parents and the world beyond the high windows we could not see out of.

Nikki continued to have his daily fits, sometimes very bad ones, during which he would shake on and on while the women held him still. Occasionally they'd take him to the dormitory after a fit, where he'd sleep for a few hours. There were also days when he'd become very aggressive if I went near him. His unpredictability was unnerving, but he was the only friend I had.

Towards the end of March, for I have the impression I had been at the asylum about two months, an opportunity presented itself for me to try to run away.

One day we were all stripped naked and taken downstairs for the weekly visit to the washroom. At the bottom of the stairs one of the boys began to scream and flail about, and two of the white-jackets grabbed him. In that brief nano-second I saw an opportunity and fled down the corridor in the opposite direction to the washroom. In hindsight it was a very stupid thing to do. I had not the faintest idea what I was going to do beyond getting away, having given no thought to the fact that I was stark naked in the middle of an institution which I did not even know *where* it was. But at the time I didn't even think of this. I just fled.

I pounded away down the corridor, the shout of one of

the women echoing in the corridor behind me. I didn't dare look back; I just focused on getting outside and away. I'd worry about practicalities like clothes later on. As I turned a corner I saw daylight ahead and, joyously, I saw that the gate had been left wide open.

In a few brief moments I was outside, and darted across the road to run through high grass between two buildings. There were shouts behind me, and not very far away either, so I ducked down behind a bush and took a quick glance behind me. I was panting hard by now as I saw three white-jackets running through the long grass. Terrified by how close they were, I darted off. I could hear their angry shouts as they spotted me.

Quite frantic by now, and on the edge of tears, I came to the end of the passageway between the two buildings, but there was no hiding place beyond, just a road between more buildings and a few parked cars. I ran across the road and hid behind a car, but the men had seen me and followed. I realised too late that they had taken either side of the cars to cut me off. I tried to dart between two cars, but the men caught up with me and grabbed me. They held me tightly and painfully by my arms and, as I sobbed, they shook me hard.

One of the men cuffed me across the head, and ignoring my noisy tears, they dragged me back along a path into the building. I was frogmarched unceremoniously down long corridors, somewhere to the back of the building, until we came to a big locked pale-blue door. It led to a dark windowless corridor of six bolted doors. The men opened a door. Inside was a bare concrete room with a small barred window set high on the wall. I became hysterical, screaming not to be put in the room, and let my legs collapse under me to drag on the floor. The men took no notice. They dragged me into the dim concrete room and dumped me on the floor; the door was slammed and bolted behind me.

I scrambled across the floor to curl up in a corner, and sobbed my heart out.

I think I spent two days locked in the isolation room, for I remember three meals were brought to me, and I spent two long terrifying nights crying in the dark, falling into exhausted sleep in the enveloping blackness.

After what seemed like an eternity, a white-jacket came and took me back to the ward. I was very subdued as I walked beside him, my arm held tightly and painfully.

On arriving at the ward I was handed over to the two women, who slammed and locked the door behind me. They gripped my arms and shook me, and it was clear they were very angry. I broke down into tears of fear.

While one woman shouted at me and slapped my head and legs, the other got a belt off the hook on the wall. I was dragged over to one of the tables and held face down across it. While one of the women held my arms, the other laid into me with the belt as hard as she could. I was now subjected to the hiding of my life, my backside and legs struck viciously hard twenty or more times. I screamed in agony.

Eventually the beating stopped, but the two women had not finished with me. As I dropped sobbing to the floor, the women got another belt off the wall with two short straps attached to it. They put it on to me as I lay on the floor, the wide waist strap buckled up tightly at the small of my back. Next my hands were pulled to my waist, and my wrists strapped and buckled to the waist-belt. In this restraint I could touch my fingers together in front of me, but apart from this small movement I could not use my hands.

Next, the women each grabbed an arm as I lay crying on the floor, and I was dragged from the day room to the empty cell, where they dumped me sobbing in fear and pain on the floor. The door was slammed shut behind me and padlocked. I was left naked and heavily restrained in the cell, empty except for a screwed-up dirty blanket in a corner. I sobbed for several hours, as much for physical pain as mental anguish. My backside and legs felt as if they were on fire. The beating had raised vivid red welts on my thighs. I dared not touch them against the floor, could not sit down, and the only position I could take for several days without agonising pain was to lie face down on the floor.

I soon became terrified that the women intended to leave me locked up just like that boy who was never let out. Food was brought to me in the cell, but because I was restrained I had to be fed by one of the women. Drinking from a cup was almost impossible, so the women placed a bowl of water on the floor, leaving me to drink like an animal.

My life became horrific. Unable to use my hands I could only curl up at night on the screwed-up blanket in the corner, and listen to the screaming of the insane boy in the next cell. I had to go to the toilet on the floor like an animal, and one of the women came in once a day to clean it away. I was soon in such a filthy and soiled state that every third day I was taken out of the cell to the washroom to be swabbed down with a wet rag and bucket of water. The isolation and loneliness were worst, and I found myself unconsciously emulating the boy in the next cell by kneeling naked on the floor in the corner, my mind numbingly empty from this mistreatment.

Nikki came occasionally and spoke to me through the bars, and I'd rush over to the door and strain, despite my restraints, to reach my fingers through the bars to touch his hands. He was my only solace in this terrible existence.

Eventually, after about a fortnight, one of the women came into the cell as I knelt huddled, my mind numb and empty, in the corner facing the wall. She unbuckled the belt, undid my wrists, and took me to the day room. It seems crazy in retrospect, but at the time I was so grateful to her for letting me loose I wanted to hug her.

In mid-April my father eventually discovered I was no longer living with my mother at Auntie Elle's house, that she'd had me committed, and I'd been in a mental institution for nearly two months.

Since September my parents' correspondence had mainly been legal letters via their lawyers. My father had tried to placate my mother, trying to get her to change her mind about the divorce, but she was adamant that she wanted a new life in Greece. My father eventually became reconciled to the divorce, so he switched tactics in March and demanded access to his children. My mother had prevaricated for several weeks until, in April, she wrote to my father that it was best if he did not have access to my sisters; she then revealed for the first time that I had gone psychotic in February and she'd had me committed to a mental institution.

My father told me later that he was horrified at this news, and immediately telephoned my mother to find out precisely what had happened and where I was. Initially my mother had refused to talk to him, but eventually she had come to the telephone. It was a fractious conversation. On several occasions tempers rose to fever pitch and they had shouted at each other down the line. However, my father persevered, for he wanted to know how ill I'd been, and where I had been sent to.

Eventually the story came out drip by drip. My mother told him that I had become mentally ill during the autumn. I had once again become very dependent, requiring a lot of care, which she and my aunts and uncles had striven to provide. However, by February I had become completely psychotic, stripping my clothes off and accusing Manolis of trying to kill me. In this completely psychotic state I had then tried to kill myself with a broken glass, slashing my face and neck, stabbing myself in the stomach. My mother justified her decision to commit me, telling my father I had been impossible to manage, and that as a psychotic autistic child this would not have happened if I'd been admitted to permanent care in Britain as she had wanted. My father demanded that he be allowed to take me out of the mental hospital and back to West Germany with him, but my mother refused his reasonable request.

After a lot of persuasion my father managed to extract from her the information that I was in the Attica State Mental Institution near Dafni, ten miles east of Athens. She went on to tell my father that she'd admitted me under her maiden name of Giorgios, and that no one except her had access to me. If my father wanted to see me, he would have to sign papers her lawyer had prepared that gave her sole custody of Vicky and Ingrid, and that he would in perpetuity pay her a substantial maintenance.

Their conversation deteriorated from there, my mother screaming abuse over the telephone before slamming the receiver down. Determined not to let the matter end like this, my father tried telephoning several more times that evening, but no one picked up the phone at Auntie Elle's.

Of course, locked away in the Attica, I was completely oblivious to my parents' bitter fight by telephone and mail. My whole environment was a locked ward where I was surrounded by fifteen severely mentally disordered and handicapped boys.

My only friend, Nikki, had not escaped this mad world. One day, when we were sitting together on the floor in the corner, the boss-eyed boy came over and lashed out at Nikki; in seconds they were rolling around on the floor fighting. Instantly the two women waded into the fight, slapping and hitting to separate them. Nikki and the other boy were dragged away and tied to cots until the following day. I'm sure that this occurred sometime towards the end of April, although of course I can't be entirely certain; I had lost track of the days. After the fight Nikki changed. He'd spend hours sitting by himself on a bench, and became very aggressive towards me if I went to him.

It was about this time that one day, after we all had our hair clipped short again, that the gowns were taken away and not returned. Apparently, now that the warmer weather had come, we were to be left naked all the time. I was mortified by this. I had tried to retain a modicum of dignity by pulling my gown about me neatly, and by this hopefully to make it clear to the women I did not consider myself mad like the others.

It was useless though, because periodically I would lapse into anguished tears at the hopelessness of my predicament, and have episodes where I would frantically beat my head against the wall. The women would wrestle me to the floor and hold me there until, sobbing, I calmed down. Now I found myself left naked like the worst of the severely defective boys, and I could tell that as I slowly deteriorated in this place so too would the differences between me and the other boys become less marked, until I would probably end up like them.

One day (I would learn later it was the beginning of May), I was kneeling in the corner of the day room when one of the white-jackets came in. He talked to the two women, who then pointed at me in the corner, and the man came over to me. Without a word, he pulled me to my feet and took me from the ward, out into the corridor and down the stairs.

I was puzzled and frightened. Had my mother forgiven me and come to take me home? Had my father come for me at last?

At the bottom of the stairs the white-jacket took me into a room full of sacks. He rummaged in a sack and produced a pair of pants, which were too big for me. Then he went to another sack and withdrew a clean gown, which he pulled on to me. Next he found a pair of sandals, again too big, which I put on.

Then, grasping me firmly by the arm, we left the building to walk in the bright sunlight down overgrown paths between buildings, along side roads, and finally into a building through a side-door, and all the time I kept hitching my pants up with one hand and slopped along in sandals that were too big for me.

The building we entered was clean and bright, with the smell of floor polish and new paint. We passed men and women who gave me no second glance. Eventually we entered a small room containing a table and two chairs. The white-jacket pushed me to sit in a chair and stood to one side. I was very puzzled, my anticipation growing that perhaps my mother, or even better my father, had come for me. I could feel a knot of anxiety growing in my stomach as I waited.

Eventually the door opened and a woman showed in a smartly dressed man in a black suit. The woman left and the man took the seat opposite me. I was really nervous by now. The man smiled at me, and to my astonishment asked how I was in English. Stunned, I was silent for a long moment.

The man reached in his jacket pocket, pulled out a bar of chocolate and handed it to me. He again asked how I was. I glanced at the white-jacket and, speaking English for the first time in months, hesitantly replied that I was okay because I was afraid of getting into trouble. It never occurred to me the white-jacket didn't understand what the black-suit or I were saying.

While I ate the bar of chocolate, black-suit explained that my father had sent him. My father could not come himself, but he had been sent to see that I was okay and being looked after.

I was utterly devastated at this revelation. After months of waiting to be rescued by my father, he had sent this man instead. The man asked again if I was being looked after. I wanted to scream this was the worst place on earth, that these people had hurt me, that I was locked up all the time with insane children. I could feel the tears welling up behind my eyes, but determined not to break down in front of this man I merely nodded and said I was okay.

A few minutes later the woman returned, and black-suit got up to leave. Before he left he turned back and, with a smile, told me not to worry. It might take a while, he said, but my father would come for me soon. Then he was gone, and I was left staring at the empty doorway.

Utterly devastated, I walked back to my building with the white-jacket. The fact that my father had sent someone on his behalf left me distraught.

Once back in the building the clothes were taken off me and, naked, I was put back in the ward with the mad children. I just curled up in a corner and could not hold on any longer. For the rest of the day I was inconsolable. Nikki came to see me, but I just pushed him away. I didn't want anyone. My father couldn't be bothered to come to see me, let alone rescue me.

I was not to know it, but my father had not been further than a single mile away from me that day. He had obtained compassionate leave from the British authorities in Germany as soon as he learnt that I was in the Attica Institution, and flown directly to Athens. Hiring a car, he had driven out to the Attica and demanded to see me. The director of the asylum consulted my file, then telephoned my mother to tell her that my father was requesting access to me, and asked was it with her permission. Knowing that my father had flown all the way from West Germany to see me, she vindictively denied him access. She told the institute director that she and my father were in the process of divorce, and that he did not have access to the children.

His hands effectively tied, the director tried to turn my father away, but he had got very angry and a furious argument developed. The director threatened to call the police, so my father had left, but immediately went to the British Embassy in Athens for help.

He telephoned someone he knew in the British Embassy in Bonn, and arranged an immediate introduction to Mr Harrison, of the Diplomatic Services Department in Athens. The Embassy in Athens now took up a role of mediation to my mother, and eventually obtained her permission for Mr Harrison – not my father – to visit me at the Attica. My father accompanied Mr Harrison, but he remained outside in the car.

Even as I was being led back to my ward, even as I sat in tears in the corner of the day room, my father and Mr Harrison were driving back to Athens, the diplomat telling my father that he was very concerned for my well-being. The way I talked and was very subdued and uncommunicative had set alarm bells ringing, and he wondered if I was indeed mentally ill.

They went to visit Dr Lumas, the British Embassy doctor. Dr Lumas had heard of the Attica. Greek mental care was among the worst in Europe in the 1970s. He told my father that I should be extricated from there as soon as possible, and taken out of Greece to where I could receive proper medical care.

That afternoon my father, Dr Lumas, and Mr Harrison drew up their campaign to have custody of me transferred from my mother to my father; it would be only then that he could get me out of the Attica. The Diplomatic Service at the Embassy would assist my father, and initiate moves to bring my case before the custody court as soon as possible. My father was advised to agree to anything my mother wanted for the moment to placate her. He was told to return to West Germany and resume his work until the wheels of the judiciary rolled and it was possible to bring my case to court.

My father reluctantly agreed to follow the advice he received from Mr Harrison. The way forward was to hire the best lawyer available, whatever the cost, and undo my mother in court. Once he had me in his hands and got me out of the country, then he could at last turn on my mother, and refuse her maintenance and challenge her for the custody of my sisters. However, there was a great deal of danger in this strategy. There was a strong chance the court might decide in my mother's favour. If that happened, then he realised I might remain locked away in the Attica for the rest of my life ...

As summer approached and the weather grew hotter, so the conditions on my ward became increasingly unpleasant. The sun streamed in through the high-set windows, turning the day room into an oven, and we children all glistened with a sheen of sweat. The windows in the day room and the dormitory were left open all the time now to give a little ventilation. The nights were just as bad because the dormitory retained the heat of the day, and it was very unpleasant trying to sleep on a rubber mattress that stuck to you when you lay down.

Trips to the washroom for the weekly hose-down with cold water were no longer an unpleasant experience, although it was always followed by a dunking in an eye- and nose-stinging bath of heavily disinfected water.

Because of the hot weather we began to get fierce thunderstorms, especially at night. I had previously liked thunderstorms, but not in a dormitory of deranged children who screamed at the top of their lungs with every flash of lightning, every thunderclap that followed. In the strobe-like flashes of lightning I could see the boys flailing about, making their metal cots rattle and shake, as they struggled against their bonds that pinned them spreadeagled upon their rubber mattresses.

It was at this time that I suffered the most horrific experience of my life. It stands alone in the horrors of my existence at the Attica Institution, and it was an experience that would leave me traumatised. It would leave me to suffer terrible nightmares throughout the rest of my childhood.

One day we were all taken off the ward, out into the corridor and downstairs to the washroom for our weekly wash. The weather by now was truly suffocating and hot, and I think it must have been early June.

At the bottom of the stairs there was a hold-up. The two women and three white-jackets pushed us boys to stand against the wall as a group of adults brought by about twenty wet, naked teenage boys. They had evidently been for their wash too that day, and seemed just as mentally disordered and impaired as the children on my ward.

It was at this moment, just as I was regarding these boys, that one of the women trod on my bare foot as she was pushing us to stand against the wall. I cried out in pain and automatically pushed at her to get her off my foot. I don't think she realised what she'd done; all she saw was a mad child making a loud noise and struggling. She grabbed me by the scruff of the neck and began hitting my head. I reacted by pulling at her arm and, not thinking about the consequences, fought back. Somehow Nikki, who was standing next to me, got caught up in the fracas, and he too found himself being slapped and pushed about.

Without thinking, and in much pain because of the way she was gripping the back of my neck, I squirmed around and bit her bare arm as hard as I could. The woman screamed, and immediately one of the white-jackets waded into the disturbance. He hit Nikki and me hard across our heads.

Without any further ado, Nikki and I were gripped by the back of our necks, given a good hard shake, and then dragged away down the corridor. As we stumbled along barefoot and naked, the man periodically kneed us from behind, as we were propelled towards the back of the building.

We eventually came to the big locked door, which led to the isolation rooms. We were bundled into the dark corridor of six bolted doors, a door was opened, and we were flung into a bare concrete room, the door slamming behind us. I heard the bolt being shot, and then the slam of the main locked door.

Distraught at the thought of being put in isolation again, and terrified of what the women would do to me on my return to the ward – my terrible beating and horrific fortnight of restraint and confinement foremost in my mind – I stood staring at the locked door, tears of anguish running down my face. I felt a hand on my shoulder, and turned to see Nikki grinning at me. It suddenly also struck me as stupid that we had been dragged away to the isolation rooms, and then locked together in the same room.

Nikki took my hands in his and giggled. He began to jump up and down and actually laughed; a rarity to hear in the Attica. Spontaneously, I too began to jump up and down; we hugged each other, a moment of closeness I had not experienced in months. This seemed to go on for ages, the sounds of our joy at being together echoing off the austere concrete walls.

Then I suddenly found myself laughing alone, for Nikki was abruptly silent, a curiously blank expression having come over his face. He seemed frozen and incapable of movement for a few seconds; then he began to tremble all over, to shiver as if from terrible cold. His eyes stared right through me as if I didn't exist. His trembles became dramatically more pronounced, until he was shaking uncontrollably as if a thousand volts of electricity were coursing through his veins. He collapsed into my arms, but he was too heavy for me to hold him, and he fell flat on his back on the concrete floor.

I immediately realised that he was having an epileptic fit. I dropped to my knees and tried to hold him still, tried to prevent him hurting himself as he flailed about and beat the back of his head on the floor. I was not strong enough. There had been many times when I had seen the two women hold Nikki still when he had a fit. They usually turned him on his side, and put him in a particular position, but I could not hold Nikki still or turn him over; he was shaking and flailing about too violently for me to handle.

His eyes were wild and staring, and he began to heave his chest up off the floor. He arched his back, plunging up and down until only his head and heels were touching the floor, his breath rasping in painful gasps. This went on and on, his arms flailing wildly. It was the most horrific thing I had ever seen in my life; his fit far, far worse that anything I had ever witnessed him have on the ward. Then he had just shaken violently all over, and the women had controlled him by placing him in a recovery position. They had known what to do. I had no idea, and what was now taking place before my terrified eyes was beyond my experience.

Suddenly Nikki's rasping breath ceased, although he continued to agonisingly arch up off the floor, his chest flexing rapidly. But there was no air entering his lungs and he was suffocating. I was not to know it at the time, but when I was older someone told me that Nikki had probably swallowed his own tongue. While it was happening I was just terrified, completely out of my depth and powerless to stop what was happening to Nikki.

As rapidly as it started, Nikki's fit ended, and he collapsed flat on the floor, his last sound a final sigh of breath escaping his lungs. He made no movement, and as I held him I suddenly realised with horror that Nikki would never move again. He was dead.

I leapt to my feet and ran to the locked door. I pounded upon it, screaming for help so loudly that what emerged was more like an animal-like scream of anguish. I pounded upon the door with my bunched fists until they began to bleed. However, I was in an isolation cell for disturbed mental patients, a cell where without doubt the inmates would often scream for help, but for help that never arrived. No one came back, and no one was interested in my screams, even if they were heard by someone in the building.

I turned back to face Nikki lying prostrate on the floor, a pale small figure that no one cared about. I went back and knelt next to him. I gathered him in my arms and, distraught, wept in a way I had never done before. I screamed in anguish, I pulled him to me and rocked his limp cool form, from which his body heat was fleeing with startling rapidity. I would never see his smile or hear his voice again. Nikki was dead, and with his death I realised for the first time how very alone I was. I cried with something akin to hysteria. The tears coursed down my face to drip on Nikki's prone form in my lap, his long dark lashes fanned across pale cheeks, his deep brown eyes never to see again.

Perhaps he was better off now. His life in this dreadful place was over. He was gone, but I was alone again. There was no one in the world I could call friend, and even my parents had left me here, abandoned and uncared for.

I wept long and hard the rest of that day, so long in fact that in the end I also wept from pain, from the ache in my arms, legs, and back, from the strain of holding Nikki to me. No white-jacket came back that day, until, in the end, I became aware that the day was drawing to a close; that the cell was becoming dark. I could not hold Nikki across my lap any longer, the strain and pain was too much for me. I tried – before the last of the daylight faded away to leave me in terrifying darkness for the night – to lay Nikki neatly on the floor. My joints were stiff from holding Nikki for hours, and I gently laid him on his back, put his arms at his side and legs together, and then I continued to kneel next to him. I held his cold hand tightly, closing his fingers about mine. I sobbed aloud through much of the night, as I knelt in the all-enveloping darkness.

With the first hints of a peach-coloured sky through the small high-set window, a new horror became apparent to me. Somehow, during the night, Nikki's eyes had opened and he stared unseeing up at the ceiling. His arm in my lap, his fingers held tightly in my hand, had become stiff, and now he gripped my hand as hard as I held his.

As a child I had no experience of death, no concept of the deathly process of rigor mortis. All I knew was that Nikki's eyes were open and he was holding my hand tightly, and I was terrified. My legs had become numb through lack of circulation, and I continued to kneel there in the first hours of a new day.

Eventually, after many hours, I heard footsteps in the corridor, the slam of a bolt, and the cell door was opened. I turned to look as a white-jacket came in. He said something in Greek, but I was too traumatised to respond, too numb to move. One glance at my tear-streaked face, at Nikki's pale body on the floor, told the man all he needed to know. He beat a hasty retreat, slamming and bolting the door again behind him.

I began to weep again, as I contemplated the fact that I was alone with a dead child. Would they think it was my fault? Would I be beaten and locked away in the cell next to the boy who was never let out, my future to be one of permanent confinement as punishment for something I had not done? I thought of all these things as I knelt on the floor with Nikki.

Suddenly there were adults in the room: two white-jackets and a woman. I was dragged away from Nikki, and dumped in the corner. I sobbed while the woman did a cursory examination on Nikki. A stethoscope was held to Nikki's chest, and the last I saw of him was when a white-jacket got me up off the floor, and took me – numb legs stumbling under me – from the room, down the corridor, and back to my ward.

I never saw Nikki again, and for some reason I was not punished by the women on the ward. I was that day dumped to sit among the severely impaired children in the middle of the room, and I continued to weep all day at the loss of my friend, distraught at the fact that I was now alone again in this dreadful place.

Following the appalling death of my only friend I began to go downhill very quickly. I had no idea of the date, but at some point June came and went, and I became eleven years old.

In early July, the weather stiflingly hot and unbearable, I began to mentally deteriorate. I began to hear a 'voice' chiding me, then my mother's voice would join in, shouting at me for hours on end. I often became so distraught I'd start beating my head against the floor, screaming at the top of my lungs. To begin with, when it did not occur so often, the two women would rush across the day room and wrestle me to the floor and pin me there until I calmed down.

However, my mental deterioration into a hallucinating state of psychosis was progressive and swift. I know I pined for Nikki dreadfully, my mind consumed with the image of his bright brown eyes staring through me to gaze unseeing at the ceiling. I had been severely traumatised by what had happened to me in that isolation cell with Nikki.

Eventually I became very mentally ill. I would sob uncontrollably for hours a day, and was put in the middle of the room with the severely mentally impaired boys where the women could more easily keep an eye on me. I would spend all day rocking, semi-catatonic, except for the periods I broke down weeping. I began to wet myself, and the difference between me and the severely impaired children was becoming less marked.

I so frequently became distraught, beating my head against the floor, that the women gave up rushing over to stop me. Their solution was to bind me to a cot all day to keep me quiet and prevent me hurting myself. Tied spreadeagled upon a rubber mattress staring at the ceiling, I sobbed and screamed, but no one ever came back. I was often bound to a cot all day, then every night as well, like the worst of the severe cases, my voice joining theirs as we screamed and cried out.

Despite my determination that I would not become like the severely disturbed boys I once pitied, I had failed and deteriorated to the point that I was as bad as the most disordered of them. In this place it was only a matter of time before a sane person could become as demented as the worst cases here.

Unbeknownst to me, my father was making great efforts to obtain custody of me, with the assistance of Dr Lumas and Mr Harrison. Every pressure was brought to bear on the

Greek authorities and my mother to ensure that my father would be granted custody of me.

The court hearing was set for 5 August 1974, and Mr Harrison wrote to my father in Germany, telling him that although the Embassy had brought a lot of pressure to bear, he should be very wary of the Greek courts. It was by no means certain the decision would go his way.

As the date got closer for the hearing, Mr Harrison again wrote to my father, telling him that they should meet on the morning of the hearing at the British Embassy, where he had organised a chauffeur-driven Embassy car that had diplomatic immunity. If the judge awarded custody to my father, they would immediately drive out to the Attica, paperwork in hand, and demand I be discharged and handed over at once, and if a reason was necessary to tell them that my father wanted me treated outside Greece.

As the day of the court hearing approached, my father left West Germany aboard a flight bound for Athens. The only thing on his mind was the thought that he might be returning in just a few days with me beside him, safe at last.

And so it happened that one hot day in August I was sitting on the floor in the middle of the day room with the severely mentally impaired boys, as they sat rocking and listening to their own voices as they made non-verbal sounds. I was terrified that if I let my guard down, my mother's voice would erupt into my head, and then she would scream and shout at me for hours. If I became distraught, beat my head on the floor to try to stop the voices, then the women would drag me off to the dormitory and tie me to a cot again. I can particularly remember that day in August as I sat on the floor trying to keep a tight rein on my mind: I mustn't think about my mother or Nikki, I told myself, and I mustn't listen to any voices that I knew could not possibly be there.

Suddenly there was a knock on the door and one of the women opened it to admit a white-jacket. They spoke briefly, before he and the woman came over and pulled me to my feet.

My mind was numb and cold by now; numb from the strain of trying to stop my mother shouting at me; left cold by the harshness of the treatment I received in this terrible place.

The man grasped me firmly by the arm and took me out of the day room, along the corridor and down the stairs. In my confused state I wondered where he was taking me.

To my surprise I was taken into the room with many sacks. The man produced an old tatty gown, which he roughly pulled on me and tied it behind my neck. This time he made no effort to find underwear or shoes for me. I was dragged barefoot back into the corridor and out through the barred gate. I now found myself taken along dusty paths between buildings under a sweltering sun. I had no idea where I was being taken.

We eventually ended up in the building with polished corridors where well-dressed men and women scurried back and forth with folders in their arms. I just gazed vaguely about me as I padded along beside the white-jacket, who had not said one word to me. We arrived at a door, which the white-jacket knocked deferentially upon. A voice answered from within, and I was ushered in.

A man with a hawkish face and glasses sat behind a large desk, and to one side stood two men. I stared at the floor. I was very frightened and had no idea what was happening. I gazed down at my bare dirty feet, then peered from under my brow across the Persian rug at the feet of the men standing to one side. I did not dare look up, but became focused on their shoes: one pair very dusty and worn, the other smart and highly polished.

There was silence for a long moment. Then a voice spoke clearly in English, the sound of his clipped accent somehow penetrating my confused mind.

'For God's sake!'

I didn't look up, so terrified was I of the four men in the room. Was I now to be punished for the death of Nikki?

As I stood staring at my feet, I suddenly became aware of something hot on my legs and a little pool of urine began to form about my feet, soaking into the rug. By now I was truly terrified. I began to shake in fear.

There were harsh words spoken between the four men, and black-shoes became very angry. I thought he was angry with me. White-jacket let go of my arm and hurried from the room. The three men began to argue, the tone of the man behind the desk wheedling and placatory, black-shoes indignant and his words heavy with anger.

After what could only have been moments the white-jacket returned and, to my surprise, began to wrap a blanket around me until I was snugly cocooned. At this point, after a few more angry words, black-shoes strode across the room and swept me off my feet. He picked me up in his arms and, with white-jacket holding the door open for him, carried me from the room, out of the building to a big black car parked in the heat of the blazing summer sun.

A chauffeur opened the back door, and black-shoes handed me in to a man sat there. Once I was in, black-shoes climbed in behind me. I kept my eyes focused on the blanket around me, and did not dare look around within the car. I just lay very still.

The chauffeur climbed in the front, started the car, and it began to move away from the front of the building down the road to the front gates. I looked out of the window. I was almost completely mentally isolated from what was happening. Black-shoes and the man were talking urgently, and the man holding me began to talk loudly, almost to shout: 'Alex! Alex! Alex! Alex!'

Some form of deep recognition of the voice entered my mind, and I looked up into the man's face. It was my father and he was crying.

It was at this point that my last reserves of self-control – of holding myself together – finally evaporated. I inhaled a deep breath until my lungs felt they would burst, then I let out a long scream at the top of my voice. It was a screech, animal-like in its ear-splitting intensity, and it went on and on. Black-shoes shouted to the chauffeur. He revved the engine hard, making the limousine leap, and charged out into the oncoming traffic. There was the squeal of braking cars and a blast of horns, then the Embassy car sped off along the road to Athens, and all the while in the back of the car I screamed and screamed, and it was unceasing and without end …

I don't remember much about the journey back to Athens that hot August day, but apparently the man who'd carried me out of the Attica was Mr Harrison, who'd come to visit me in April. I had not recognised him. During the journey, while I screamed unendingly like a completely demented thing, he used the car telephone to ring Dr Lumas. My father and Mr Harrison, horrified by the terrible state I was in, realised they could not take me to my father's hotel, so they took me directly to Dr Lumas's house.

All I vaguely remember was the car sweeping up a driveway to a big white house. The car stopped, and my father hurriedly carried me up the steps and in through the front door, and all the time I kept emitting an ear-piercing shriek, a continuous feral scream of mental pain and anguish.

I was dumped on the floor, the blanket was pulled off me, and Dr Lumas gave me an injection in the arm to sedate me. That was the end of my day; I don't remember anything more.

When I eventually woke up, I was snug and warm in a bed, and my father was seated on a chair next to me. He spoke to me, but I couldn't understand anything he said. I began to sob, but at least my need to emit my demented screams of anguish had passed.

I was later to learn, one day in the future when I was old

enough to understand, that when my father got me back I was mentally shattered, with pronounced hysteria, psychosis, severe malnutrition, rampant scabies and, at the age of eleven, I weighed under four stone.

Later that morning Dr Lumas came to see me. After a cursory examination he gave me another injection to keep me calm. Then my father pulled some new clothes on me. Black-suit – Mr Harrison – appeared, and talked to me, telling me I was going to be all right now, but it was very important I stayed calm; this my father repeated while stroking my head and patting my hand.

I was so sleepy I could not keep awake, and found myself carried by my father out of the room, down the stairs, and out to the big Embassy car. Everyone clambered aboard, and we set off for Athens airport.

I slept most of the time, even in the airport when my father carried me while Mr Harrison held his holdall. There was a brief delay while someone in a uniform was summoned to check the papers, then we miraculously passed through passport control. Because I had only been listed on my mother's passport, Mr Harrison had arranged a diplomatic passport for my father by virtue of his role with the British authorities in West Germany. My name had been entered on this diplomatic passport, and it was more than any mere passport control officer at Athens's Eleniko Airport dared risk to challenge such an important travel document.

We left Athens that afternoon aboard a West Germany-bound Lufthansa flight, with me sleeping across two seats;

my head and shoulders safely cradled in my father's arms. Once or twice a stewardess came with soft drinks for me, and I, very drowsy, would rouse myself to drink. But I was so heavily sedated that I was barely conscious and soon fell asleep again. And all the time the plane sped across Europe, leaving Greece far behind.

My father had, after months of delay, successfully rescued me from an appalling mental institution, but the big question that preyed on his mind as he held me and we flew ever westward – the distance between the plane and Athens growing by the minute – was how much damage had been done to me, and would I ever recover?

CHAPTER 8

Germany

I gazed out of the first-floor window down into the street, and watched as men in khaki uniforms sauntered past. Occasionally the passing of an army Land Rover would pique my interest, and I'd press my forehead against the cool glass to watch it until it passed out of sight around the corner.

I spent most of my days standing at this window in the lounge of my father's flat at the military base north-west of Cologne. It was a comfortable flat, with nice furniture and a television in the corner. On the coffee table were comics and colouring books, which I had no interest in. I wandered the flat all day like an embodied wraith, an insubstantial being that was a mere shadow of my former self. My nights were truly terrible. Every night I had appalling nightmares that left me screaming and sobbing, and had my father rushing into my room to comfort me.

My father, and a nice lady called Marilyn from the flat next door, took it in turn to stay with me all the time. They were particularly tuned-in to prevent me becoming upset, when I would break down in hysterical tears, falling to the floor and beating my head against the carpet. Then they would pounce on me, and hold me still until I calmed down again. Dad would sit all day with a newspaper, keeping a sly eye on me as I wandered the flat, always eventually returning to the window, where I'd rest my forehead against the cool glass, and watch the outside world.

I was mentally shattered – my experiences in the Attica Institution had all but destroyed me – and it remained to be seen whether I would ever recover. I did not want to talk. In my traumatised state I was utterly consumed by the appalling experiences of what I had suffered in the Attica and the loss of Nikki, whom I mourned so deeply.

On arriving at the base in the evening after our flight from Athens, my father had immediately telephoned a doctor, who came to the flat to see me. He had tut-tutted as he examined me and placed a cold stethoscope on my painfully thin frame. All through this examination I had shaken in fear, and when he talked to me, asked me questions, I had stuttered a brief answer, my few words stumbling from lack of use. I had barely spoken a word during my last six months at the Attica Institution; indeed, I'd hardly been permitted to talk in English for five months at Auntie Elle's house. The doctor prescribed a number of tablets, and a disgusting white cream in which I had to be covered from head to foot in cure the scabies I had caught in the Attica.

Despite my poor physical condition, the greatest concern was for my mental well-being. I was in a truly terrible state. I could hardly talk. I stuttered dreadfully, hesitated over every word, and was terrified of giving the wrong answer. The result: I refused to talk at all unless given no alternative.

The day after my arrival at the base a psychiatrist came to the flat who, with my father sitting to one side, sat with me at the table and asked me all sorts of searching questions.

Did I have bad dreams? Was I frightened in the day, and if so what of? Did I hear voices? Was my memory playing tricks on me? Did images and memories of bad things from my time at the Attica flash into my mind and upset me?

These were the general vein of questions asked, and as I stuttered my answers it became apparent that I was not at all well. In the end I broke down in anguished tears, sobbing hysterically, and the psychiatrist had to abandon his examination.

His diagnosis was that I had been severally traumatised by my experiences at the Attica, and was likely to be suffering from a condition called post-traumatic stress disorder (PTDS). Far worse, he believed I was suffering a psychotic illness again. He told my father that my experiences in Greece had tipped me over the precipice into these two severe mental illnesses, and that one exacerbated the other. In his opinion the place for me was in hospital care.

Naturally my father was very upset by this diagnosis. He had managed to take nearly two weeks off work on compassionate grounds, but his work was important and he could not stay at home permanently to look after me. During a long discussion with the psychiatrist, my father reluctantly decided I needed more care than he was capable of providing. I needed to be in hospital.

In the meantime, the psychiatrist provided my father with a prescription for a number of drugs, primarily sedatives and the anti-psychotic, Chlorpromazine. The psychiatrist told my father to leave the matter to him, and he would locate a suitable German facility for mentally ill children to which I could be admitted.

It was a bright summer's day as we sped along in my father's new car. While I had been in Greece my father had sold the motorhome. There had been a captain at the base who was being posted to Hong Kong. This army officer had just bought a new red Rover P6 3500, which he couldn't take with him, so he sold it to my father.

Now we travelled through the German countryside, my father's attention on the road while he talked. As for me, my mind wandered as I gazed out of the window at the passing villages and towns. I was not at all well and I frequently broke down in tears for no obvious reason that my father could tell. I knew full well what the reason was. I was suffering repeated horrible flashbacks of the Attica Institution, and I could hear my mother shouting at me, but I dared not tell him this.

That Friday morning my father told me that we were going away for the weekend. He had placed two holdalls in the car boot, and we set off from the base. All the while we travelled my father talked incessantly, trying to keep my mind off things that upset me. We counted Volkswagen Beetles. He chatted about his work. He talked about my grandparents. Always a constant stream of conversation that I found hard to keep up with. It was basically one-sided; I just huddled up on the seat, feet up, knees tucked under my chin, and gazed out of the window at the passing countryside.

Eventually we arrived at a small German town called Wetter in Westphalia, about 60 miles from the base. My father proceeded to negotiate turns and junctions until we came to a big building that I took to be the hotel. I looked up at the big country house while my father parked the car.

As soon as we entered the building I was immediately suspicious. I didn't have much experience of hotels, but this didn't look like one. It had the austere practical look – polished floors and painted walls – of a hospital. My father closed the front door behind us and, as I turned back from him, I was absolutely horrified to see a nurse and doctor in a white lab-coat coming down the corridor.

With sudden sick realisation I knew that my father had brought me to a hospital of some kind. Was I being abandoned in one of these places again? I fell to the floor and clutched my father's legs, screaming and sobbing to him not to leave me here. Within moments there were several nurses holding me, trying to calm me down. But I could not be consoled. I sobbed hysterically.

I was lifted up off the floor, and two nurses held me in a chair while my father talked at length to an elderly man. My father then turned his attention to me, and knelt so that he was on my level. Holding my hands in his, he explained that I was very ill and needed proper care, which these nice people would give me. I wasn't going to be here long, he promised, just until I was well again. I took no notice of his placatory words. I just sobbed and screamed, struggling against the nurses to get free and run away.

At this moment I spotted a nurse hurrying over with a shiny kidney dish. She handed something to the elderly man, and before I could react he gave me an injection in my arm. Within moments I felt very sleepy, and my last memory of that traumatic day is of my father holding my hands with tears in his eyes.

I can see now that it must have been a terrible thing for my father to take me to this mental hospital for children in Westphalia. He had to deceive me to get me there, knowing that I would react very badly at the prospect of being placed in another psychiatric unit. However, I don't think he fully realised the implications for me. In my terror at being brought here all I could think was that I was being abandoned again, this time by my father.

The staff at the Wetter Institute for Children with Mental Illness were very kind to me, but I was a difficult patient. In my traumatised state I withdrew into myself and refused to have anything to do with anyone, despite the fact it was a very well run and comfortable unit for mentally troubled children.

On the my first night the staff put me in a room with a

boy of my own age. However, this proved to be a disaster because I awoke repeatedly all through the night screaming and sobbing because of my nightmares and flashbacks. The next morning a kind nurse named Fräulein Hepp arranged for me to have a room of my own, where she installed a table lamp with a dim bulb that could be left on all night.

Having a night-light in my room helped me significantly. I continued to have very troubled nights with horrific nightmares, but when I awoke in the light I could relate to the room, to my surroundings, and knew I was safe and not in the Attica.

Regardless of more stable nights, it only took a few days for my psychiatrist, Dr Nordbusch, to realise that I was actually declining. A hospital environment seemed to exacerbate my condition. Every day for the first week I had sessions with Dr Nordbusch, who tried to get me to talk. It was not something I could, aged eleven, articulate in words, and I did not want to talk about it. I just broke down in tears and the daily sessions always had to be abandoned because I became so distressed. Indeed, I suffered such frequent upsets and disturbances that Dr Nordbusch decided that he'd have to try something different. He came to the conclusion that it was not beneficial for me to stay at the Wetter Institute, regardless of how understanding the staff were to me.

A week after I had been admitted to the hospital my father drove to Wetter and met with Dr Nordbusch. He told my father I was very troubled. The psychosis, which he believed was not too severe and could be brought under control with drugs, was not his primary concern. He was much more concerned by my flashbacks and nightmares, the post-traumatic stress disorder. He said that I was very mentally disturbed with memories that, unless treated, could eventually cause catastrophic psychological damage. I was like a pressure-cooker on a stove, which, unless the heat was reduced, would blow its safety valve. If this happened, then I'd collapse into a state of severe mental illness, complete with chronic psychosis, from which I might never recover. If that were to happen at the tender age of eleven, then I might become so severely traumatised that I could end up under psychiatric care for the rest of my life. It was therefore a race against time to find the best treatment for me – to release my safety valve – before I suffered a complete mental breakdown. My father described my screaming fit on his rescuing me from the Attica, and Dr Nordbusch confirmed this was just the sort of reaction he feared. In my precarious mental state I could collapse like that again at any moment.

Dr Nordbusch told my father that he had an idea. There was a clever and skilled psychologist named Dr Edgar Schultz, who lived only 20 kilometres away in the small town of Hagen. If Dr Schultz was willing to take the case on, then he suggested that I be sent to live with him and his wife at his house for a few weeks. Out of a hospital environment I might well improve, and Dr Schultz could conduct counselling that would gently let me release my 'safety valve' in a controlled and safe manner. However, the doctor warned, Dr Schultz was a specialist, and as such he charged

a significant fee. My father told the doctor that whatever Dr
Schultz's fee was it would be met.

And so it was that, after a stay at the Wetter Institute of
only ten days, a kindly old man with a big moustache and
white hair came and talked to me. After a brief conversation,
during which I had stuttered and shaken in fear, he asked if
I would like to go and live in his house with him and his
wife for a few weeks. With the thought of being offered a
chance to leave hospital, and much taken with Dr Schultz's
soft voice and evident kind nature, I stuttered out an affirm-
ative reply. The old man smiled at me and nodded his head,
and said that I could leave that same afternoon to go and
live in his house.

To my immense joy, that same afternoon, my holdall on
the back seat of a battered old white Volkswagen Beetle, I
left the Wetter Institute with Dr Schultz, my destination the
small Westphalian town of Hagen.

Dr Schultz lived in a smart residential street of large
detached houses. As soon as we arrived, Frau Schultz
emerged from the kitchen in a flour-covered apron, and
made me very welcome. Her English was not as good as Dr
Schultz's, but she made great efforts to speak English to me,
laughing and pinching my thin cheek as she spoke.

I immediately felt safe with Dr Schultz, especially when
he took me upstairs and showed me a big bedroom that was
to be mine. A table lamp had been placed in the room in
anticipation of my arrival.

Late that afternoon Dr Schultz took me outside where he
opened a shed door and took out two bicycles: his own, an

old-fashioned bike, and a smaller child's bike, which was his grandson's. Then, to my surprise, he directed me to take the bike out into the tree-lined street, and we set off along the pavement, heading towards the town centre.

Dr Schultz took me into Hagen, where he bought vegetables in the market for the evening meal, placing them in his panniers, then took me into the dim interior of a beautiful church of which he was greatly proud.

We returned to his home and sat in his study, making gentle conversation, mostly, I have to say, from him. At six, he, Frau Schultz and I sat in the big kitchen for the evening meal. It was a very Germanic sort of meal, with much red cabbage, potatoes, and meat.

And so my first day with the Schultzes ended, and at nine in the evening I was given my tablets and sent to bed, the table lamp left on for me all night.

That night Dr Schultz discovered for the first time how troubled I really was. I woke up screaming and sobbing at one in the morning, and became very upset indeed. Dr Schultz immediately came to see me, to try to comfort and support me, but instead of making a big deal of the situation, he calmly suggested that I lie down and try not to become too deeply engrossed in my memories. He told me to try and let go of the bad memories; they were only that – memories – and I couldn't be hurt by them. He sat with me through the remainder of that first night, and when I awoke, which happened several times, he was always at my bedside, book in hand, ready to talk to me and support me if I needed it.

I spent a month with Dr Schultz and his wife, Gertrud. It was without a doubt the safest and happiest I had felt for years. Every Sunday my father came to visit me, laden with a bag containing dozens of Mars bars in the hope that if I ate them all I would put some badly needed weight back on. He'd spend the whole day with me and was made welcome by Dr Schultz and his wife, eventually leaving after the evening meal for the long drive back to the base.

At this time my father was also pleased by the way his work was winding up in Germany. As a result of reduced East–West tension, he was told in September that his services would be dispensed with in October and he could return to civilian life as a lecturer in Britain. He therefore made plans to return to Britain and, while I was living with Dr Schultz in Hagen, popped back to Wales to make arrangements for our return home.

He had spoken at length to Dr Schultz in early October, and was told by the psychologist that, although I was still far from well, my time of mental crisis had passed. Although I still had severe PTDS, and probably a form of mild psychosis, which the drugs had under control, in his opinion I could now return to live a normal life at home with him.

I was still far from fully recovered, and it would be months before I would be mentally fit enough to attend school, but Dr Schultz felt that all I needed now was time and care for my psychological wounds to heal. This would likely take months, perhaps even years.

During my time with Dr Schultz, I had undergone a difficult healing process. We had sat for two hours every morning while he talked to me; got me to talk to him about the things that had happened to me, and that had been very difficult. Although I still suffered nightmares and intrusive flashbacks about my time in Attica, I would have to learn to live with these memories; they would be with me for the rest of my life. I also discovered that Dr Schultz did not merely believe that my time in the Attica was all that troubled me. He went to great lengths to try to explain to me that what my mother had done to me was just as cruel as the things that had happened at the Attica.

I still deeply mourned the loss of Nikki, but, explained Dr Schultz, his death had not been my fault. I should never have been placed in the situation with Nikki to start with. During these sessions about Nikki I became terribly distressed, and it was sometimes very hard for Dr Schultz to console me. But he had persevered, and eventually I understood that I was not responsible for the death of my friend.

Eventually, after four weeks' intensive therapy with Dr Schultz, it became clear that I had turned a corner. My mental time bomb had been slowly defused. I continued to have nightmares, and would need to sleep in the light for years to come as a sort of grounding-rod to pull me back from my memories, which were often so powerful that I could forget I was now safe.

On the last evening of my stay with Dr Schultz, his wife made a big cake and prepared a special dinner to celebrate my departure the following day. That evening we all sat down to a four-course dinner of Westphalian delicacies. I went to bed that evening happier than I had been for years. I lay in bed that evening, thinking of life with my father, the glow from the table lamp throwing the room into strange comforting shadows, and eventually fell asleep.

The journey from West Germany and across northern France took most of the day, as I sat next to my father in his Rover P6 as he sped at nearly 90 miles per hour along autobahns and French motorways. I listened to the engine growl as we quickly ate the miles away heading towards Calais, to cross the Channel back to Britain.

There was a brief rainstorm in northern France, lightning glimpsed on the horizon as we sped ever westward, the wipers flicking back and forth as I watched the raindrops running up the windscreen, the flow of wind strong enough to force the rain into a gravity-defying dance on the glass.

My father had collected me from the Wetter Institute only the day before. I had been there a week after Dr Schultz had returned me for a mental assessment by Dr Nordbusch. I was much changed since he had last seen me. I was still unstable with a terrible uncertainty and stutter that dogged my daily life, but at least I was more accepting of my situation, and not prone to episodes when I would flop on the floor sobbing.

I was, however, still subject to spontaneous flashbacks that upset me. But, as Dr Schultz and Dr Nordbusch explained to my father, I had somehow survived the most terrible experiences. I had experienced and seen things at the Attica that no eleven-year-old should ever have to live with.

My father stopped in Calais town centre for a wander and a drink. He deftly parked the car and after a trip round the shops, we stopped at a bar. Here, despite the overcast afternoon sky, the hint of rain to come, we sat outside; I with a Coca-Cola, he with a cigar and a glass of Pernod, as we watched the traffic passing by. It was so different to my existence of just two months ago, where I had been locked away and all but forgotten in what seemed to me the worst place on earth.

I found I had to keep doing a double take of my surroundings to pull myself back to the present. I had to let go of the past. I resisted the temptation to cry, blinking back tears, and forced myself to stutter a question to my father, asking him why could we not stay in Calais for a few days?

My question seemed to bring my father back from his reverie. He looked at me and smiled. He reached across the table and patted my hand. 'No,' he told me. 'It's time we finished our drinks. It's time to go home …'

In less than an hour we were aboard a battered old ferry with rust disgorging from its seams like an overstuffed toy, and the crossing passed all too quickly before we were back in Britain, back to a land where everyone drove on the left of the road, back where I could read road and shop signs, and understood what they meant. It was comforting to be home at last. I watched my father as he gunned the P6 up the steep road out of Dover, rapidly overtaking cars and lorries that struggled against the steep gradient. My father's car ate up the miles as we headed along the A2, signs declaring the direction to be Canterbury and London.

After passing through Canterbury, my father suddenly pulled the car over into a lay-by on the brow of a hill. He told me to get out of the car and we stood together gazing at the countryside. A thrush chirped in the bushes, its last song of the day before what promised to be a wet night.

My father just stood gazing at the Kent countryside, the sun setting in a vivid scar on the western horizon. I stood before him watching the sunset and feeling the comforting weight of his hands upon my shoulders. I was safely back in Britain, and safe with my father. I could feel my tears welling up behind my eyes. I tried terribly hard to hold them back. I did not want to cry, not now. Now was a time of happiness, a time of relief that I was safe.

In the end I could not hold back any longer, and broke down in tears. I shook and shook as I was racked by deep drawn sobs. But they were not tears of sadness. They were tears of relief. I was back in Britain, and back with my father. He held me as I cried, and I thought he would never let go. Whatever happened from now on, I knew that my father would be there to protect me. It was a time to let go of the past, a time to look forward to the future.

CHAPTER 9

Lull Before the Storm

'We commit the body of our brother here departed ...' intoned the vicar as I stood beside my father in the cold November rain.

I gazed into the muddy hole into which rivulets of water poured down from the surrounding soil into the water-logged grave. To my left my grandmother was sobbing, bolstered by my father's arm. The men of the funeral directors had just lowered my grandfather's coffin into the grave. The women standing around the grave all wept during the proceedings.

My father had not been there for his parents in their time of need, during the last months working in West Germany. He had only managed to visit them once during the four months between my grandfather's diagnosis of lung cancer, the futile attempts at treatment, and the terrible end when hope was extinguished and he finally died.

The vicar began to conclude the service: 'Earth to earth; ashes to ashes; dust to dust ...'

It was so final when everyone turned away from the hole

in the ground, and slowly walked away; back to the funeral limousines that would take us to my Uncle Tom's house for a cup of tea and a piece of cake.

My father and I had been back in Britain a week, our arrival at my grandparents' house in Cardiff so ill timed that we arrived the same evening my grandfather died. I arrived full of happiness at being with my father straight into a house of mourning. Auntie Pat and Uncle Tom (Dad's brother) were there to console my grandmother. We arrived at her semi-detached house in the quiet leafy suburb of Fairwater just three hours after they had been with my grandfather when he died in hospital.

Despite her trauma that day, the sight of me gave my grandmother new purpose.

She was horrified at my condition, the fact I weighed less than four stone, was pale and trembled at the slightest unexpected sound. It made her determined to take me in hand.

My grandmother bustled about in the kitchen making me an omelette. I stood by the door, watching her and straining to listen to my father in the sitting room as he, in murmured tones, told my uncle and aunt of my fragile mental state, the story of how my mother had nearly got me killed.

My father did not want to take me back to our home in Cornwall. It had too many painful memories, and he was determined to make a fresh start in South Wales. He had obtained a university position as a senior lecturer in politics and economics. In the months and years ahead, as he began to be consulted on Middle Eastern affairs, this would become of increasing importance to his career and my future.

The house was large with high gables, and a long drive that swept up the side to twin garages at the rear, the front and rear gardens full of lush bushes.

My father smiled at me as he opened the front door.

We had been back in Britain for three weeks. It was now late November and this was the tenth house we had been to view. My father was not due to take up his university post until January, so he had the rest of the autumn and early winter to find us a house in Cardiff. His search concentrated in the suburb of Fairwater, not far from my grandmother's house.

We were still living in my grandmother's house at this time, and she had by now seen and heard for herself my terrible nightmares, my periods of disorientation when I suffered flashbacks, and needed a lot of support to stop me becoming hysterical.

That November morning turned out to be a defining moment, for the instant we stepped over the threshold into the deserted house, it became clear to me that this would be home. It was a large 1930s property with entrance hall, three reception rooms, a large kitchen and dining area, and a conservatory. Upstairs, the house had a wide bright landing leading to five bedrooms, and an old-fashioned bathroom.

On the basis of his substantial salary from the university, my father bought the house in early December 1974.

There then followed three weeks while workmen redecorated the house and installed a new bathroom suite. I rarely went to the house at this time. I stayed with my grandmother, while my father supervised the builders in renovating the house.

Because the only clothes I possessed were virtually what I stood up in, my grandmother took pleasure in taking me into the city centre on the bus several times a week to go shopping for clothes. As a treat, every time we went into town she took me to a smart restaurant called the Louis that served coffee and a silver platter of cream cakes between ten and noon. Then, after a morning's browsing of the high street and department stores, we returned at 1.30 p.m. to a reserved table at the Louis for lunch.

I was a fragile child, small, underweight, looking at most about nine or ten years old, not my true age of eleven and a half. However, these trips were therapeutic for both my grandmother and me. For despite my panic attacks, which were very upsetting, I was gradually being integrated back into the normal world. For my grandmother, I believe these days out gave her renewed purpose after the death of my grandfather. They had been devoted to each other for forty-four years, and I frequently found her weeping quietly to herself in her kitchen. I would just go and hug her. I didn't need to say anything. It was my only way to thank her for all she was doing for me.

It was a bright February morning when my father took me to Kings School Cardiff. I had not been to school since

November 1972. It was now February 1975, and I had not had any education at all for nearly two and a half years.

Kings specialised in the education of children who had minor learning or behavioural problems. It predominantly provided education for 'difficult' children, who it had been considered would struggle in secondary school. However, Kings, set in a very big house off Newport Road, was private and expensive. It was a boys-only school for 250 pupils aged eleven to sixteen years, with uniform of blazer and grey trousers.

On my first day at school I was very nervous indeed. My new teacher, Mr Channon, was a kindly old man, and not scathing about my educational limitations. On the first day he patiently sat with me as I struggled to read to him; he then asked me basic maths questions, which I tried unsuccessfully to answer. It was soon evident to Mr Channon that I was very far behind my peers, even in his class of educationally challenged children.

There were three classes per year at Kings. 'A' was for the bright pupils. Next came the 'B's, who were not so intellectually gifted. The last third of pupils made up the 'C's who were problematic to teach. 'C's – or 'the clay class' as was the common banter among the boys in the playground – were of very limited ability.

Because of my father's work, he only managed to take me and collect me from school every day for the first week. After this initial phase he made arrangements for a taxi to return me to my grandmother's house every afternoon, from where he collected me at 6 p.m.

However, these arrangements were not to last long.

After I had been at Kings a fortnight, the headmaster made a suggestion to my father. There was a boy at Kings of my age in 1B called Paul Nutt. Paul was dyslexic and known to all as 'Peanut' because his name was P. Nutt. He too lived in the suburb of Fairwater, just a few streets from my house. His mother was having problems taking Peanut to and from school because she was a divorcee with a part-time job. Mr Beavan, the headmaster, suggested to my father that he and Mrs Nutt split the school-run between them.

My father immediately came to an arrangement with Margaret Nutt to pool their efforts, he from now on taking me and Peanut to school in the mornings, while she would collect us in the afternoon. I then stayed at Peanut's house until 6 p.m., when my dad returned from the university to collect me.

As I suppose was bound to happen, Margaret and my father began to get very friendly, and as a foursome we began to do things together on weekends. On Saturdays my father took us all to the nearby seaside town of Penarth, with its Victorian pier and promenade that had a selection of cafés, where we had lunch. On Sundays, Margaret would cook lunch, following which we went to Roath Park for a walk around the large boating lake.

Peanut soon began calling my father 'Uncle Peter', and I found myself calling his mother 'Auntie Margaret'. A relationship was beginning to develop between my father and Margaret, and I became very fond of the pleasant woman with short brown hair who collected Peanut and me from school every day. I had never had a genuinely kind 'motherly figure' in my life before. My own mother had hated me and treated me very badly for as long as I could remember. I suppose as any child has needs and looks for affection where it can get it, I began to transfer affection to Margaret Nutt.

However, life was about to throw a spanner in the works in a way that I never believed would happen. My father began to be consulted on Middle Eastern affairs, and what subsequently occurred initiated an extended chain of events that would ultimately place me in peril.

My father was an expert on East–West relations and the Middle East. At the beginning of May 1975, he was contacted by the office of the Israeli Prime Minister. The Israelis wanted someone to act as an unofficial emissary to the Syrians and Egyptians.

In my father the Israelis saw a man who had an in-depth knowledge of Soviet foreign policy and Middle Eastern politics. A neutral intermediary who could go to Damascus in an unofficial capacity to open the first tentative diplomatic talks with the Syrians on making the Yom Kippur War ceasefire into something more permanent. Negotiations with the Egyptians were to take place at a later date.

And so it was that I found myself left for ten days to stay with my grandmother, while my father flew to the Middle East. Before he left my father had been careful to explain to me that his work was taking him away from me again for a short time. He had drawn up an itinerary for me that included school days and a trip out on the first weekend with my grandmother. On the second weekend he even agreed that I could stay at Peanut's house, a ten-minute walk from my grandmother's house two streets away.

My father left on the first Thursday in May 1975 to drive to Heathrow and take his flight to Tel Aviv.

I found the first weekend with my grandmother very boring. We went into the city centre on the Saturday, but as a child of nearly twelve years I was outgrowing the time when I was content to stay with my grandmother and wander the shops with her. I wanted to be more adventurous, and I wanted to spend more time with my friend Peanut.

I was much happier on the second weekend when, collected from school with Peanut by Margaret, we stopped briefly at my grandmother's house for me to change out of my school uniform. My grandmother and Margaret fell into an easy relationship, for while I went upstairs to change I could hear them chatting in the hall downstairs. I stopped changing at one point and stood on the landing listening as my grandmother talked about how proud she was of her son the academic. Then she dropped her voice to a murmur, but I could still hear her telling Margaret about the dreadful mistake he had made in marrying my mother, who had hated me and nearly killed me. For some reason I was really furious with my grandmother for disclosing that. My past wasn't something my father or I had ever talked about to Margaret.

'Of course Alex's not well you know,' I heard my grandmother confide. 'His mother damaged him and I'm sure Peter and I don't know how far that damage runs. We just hope he never becomes mentally ill again.'

Fuming, I finished dressing, and made a point of slamming the bedroom door. The conversation downstairs was instantly cut off as if it had never happened, and I clattered down the stairs, holdall in hand.

My grandmother was all solicitude as she bent to kiss me goodbye. I didn't return her kiss. I just went over to Margaret and Peanut who stood in the hall, and said I was ready to go.

We three got into Margaret's Mini for the run up the road to her house, and as we drove away my grandmother waved to me. I just nodded, still quietly fuming at her. I was very wary that Friday evening with Margaret, but she gave no sign that she knew my secret, showed no sign that she didn't like me any more.

I returned to my grandmother's house on Sunday afternoon after a wonderful weekend with Peanut, and knowing that my father was due home late that night. I badgered my grandmother to let me stay up to await his arrival, but she told me he would not be back until after midnight. I went to bed at 9.30 p.m. and tried to stay awake, listening for the telltale bang of the front door that would herald my father's return, but I never heard it for I soon fell into my usual fitful sleep.

On the following morning I got up to get ready for school, and found my father in the sitting room, cup of coffee in hand. I flew across the room to hug him, full of excited chatter about all that I had done in the last ten days, and went to school happy in the knowledge that my father and I would be home that evening.

It took several days for me to broach the subject, but before the next weekend when we were expected to go to my grandmother's house for tea on Saturday, I told my father that I'd heard my grandmother telling Margaret about Mum and my mental problems. My father said nothing, but I saw by the set of his face that he was very angry.

We went to my grandmother's that Saturday, but we left early, and as we went I could see on my grandmother's face that she thought she'd unwittingly offended my father in some way. I felt very sorry indeed for her, and despite my indignation at her spilling of my secrets to Margaret, I wished I had not told my father. Now, aged nearly twelve, I had learnt an important lesson. If ever I was in such a position again, I told myself, I would keep my feelings to myself. My past, and its repercussions, were subjects I could not discuss with my father, not for years to come, but by then it would be far too late.

It was May and the summer began to make itself felt with hotter and sunnier days. I became increasingly excited that it would soon be my twelfth birthday on 7 June. I had missed my previous two birthdays, and that was something that was irreplaceable.

By the end of May I became aware that my father and grandmother were having secret conversations. As I played in my grandmother's back garden on Saturday afternoons, I could see them talking by the French doors, with furtive glances in my direction. If I went into the house, their conversation suddenly died, and there would be embarrassed coughs, and the strands of some mundane conversation would pick up:

'... and as I was saying to Mrs Campbell ...' my grandmother would begin.

I could tell something was up, and I became convinced they were plotting some wonderful surprise for my twelfth birthday, which was the following Saturday. I let my father have his secret plans, and did not ask any questions. At last the week passed. For a change – which was highly significant as far as I was concerned – my father arranged with Margaret that *he* would collect me from school that Friday afternoon.

Finally, it was 3.30 Friday afternoon and I flew out of school to where my father sat in his car. It was going to be my birthday tomorrow, and by now I had convinced myself that something wonderful was afoot.

My father smiled at me as I clambered into the car, and began to talk to me in his usual way as he drove, his eyes playing on the road ahead. The conversation slowly began to turn to my problems over the last few years. How I had survived them, and how it was important for me to put those things behind me. Then he began to say he had a surprise for me at home; but, he emphasised, it was all right if I was a bit startled to begin with. The important thing, he repeated, was now that I was twelve I should not let the past play on my mind. I didn't understand that. I let it pass, and the conversation moved on while my father told me that the future would be different from now on.

We arrived home, and by now I was utterly convinced he had bought me a dog, for I had been pestering him for weeks that we should get a puppy.

I watched eagerly as my father turned the key in the lock; the front door swung open, and we hurried in. He put his hand on my shoulder and smiled at me as he opened the drawing room door and ushered me in.

I heard a cough and saw a sudden movement. There was a blonde woman in the room with her back to me. I watched her as, almost as if in slow motion, she stood up from the sofa, a young child in her arms, and turned to face me. The sunlight streamed in through the bay window to reflect off her glasses, giving her a strange inhuman quality.

I stood stunned and rooted to the spot as if poleaxed under the steady gaze of the woman I had not seen in a year and a half.

No one said a word for a long, eternal, moment.

'Hello, Alex,' my mother said at long last.

The room began to wax and wane, to sway from side to side, and I collapsed in a dead faint …

CHAPTER 10

A Sense of Déjà vu

The hands that held my shoulders and propelled me along shook me savagely, and I, terrified, cried out for them to leave me alone. The corridor before me seemed endless; in the distance I could see the pale-blue locked door.

The door opened and gaped before me.

I screamed, yet still the shaking of my shoulders continued. From somewhere far away I could hear my name being called.

I opened my eyes, and looked at my father in his dressing gown, holding me by my shoulders.

He had awoken me from my nightmare.

I looked over my father's shoulder, and saw my mother standing by my bedroom door. I knew by her expression that I was no longer safe. There was a malevolent force in my home that hated me, and I was terrified …

During my father's trip to Israel in May he had visited my mother in Athens to try and salvage their marriage.

When my father told me this I was flabbergasted. Despite knowing that my mother hated me, despite knowing that she had mistreated me in Greece and nearly got me killed, despite her months of intransigence in her demands for a divorce, my father had made one last offer of peace to her, and they had become reconciled. They had decided to give their marriage one last go.

In retrospect I don't think my mother wanted to return to Britain. She had no choice, because by May 1975 her money had run out, together with her welcome at Auntie Elle's. My father had a good career, a nice house, and a high standard of living, whereas my mother was in Greece with two children and fast becoming insolvent. Solution: return to my father in Britain, who was willing to forgive anything to get his daughters back. Vicky was now aged eleven, and Ingrid had turned two.

Years later my father told me that *I* had been the biggest hurdle to overcome. My mother had insisted that *if* she was to return to Britain with my sisters, he would have to agree that *she* take all the care decisions regarding me. If I became mentally ill again, then that was it. Their marriage, she claimed, had almost floundered because of the strain of looking after me when I had been psychotic. If I became mentally ill again, then I would have to be admitted to hospital care.

Despite knowing my mother had taken me to the brink of destruction, my father was so overwhelmed by the thought he could get my sisters back that he agreed to all my mother's conditions. My mother was always very convincing, and many years later my father told me he had been persuaded by her argument that I'd caused the problems in the family – difficult for any family to cope with – and it was that that had almost caused their marriage to fail. My mother told him she would give their marriage a second chance, but that she was not prepared to let my mental problems cause upheaval in the home again. It was to be a recipe for disaster. Once again I had been sacrificed in my father's desire for family unity.

Within a few days of my mother's return, my father had fallen completely under her spell again. It has to be said that when she wanted, my mother could be charming, with a winning smile and a delightful laugh.

I wasn't fooled for a moment.

By the weekend following her return my father was very pleased with himself, and hinting at a surprise for my mother on Saturday morning. The 'surprise' turned out to be a new maroon Triumph Herald estate. Naturally my mother was delighted. It won my father a hug, and then she excitedly sat in the driver's seat and fiddled with all the controls.

This was one of the few pleasant moments of my mother's return, for there were far less agreeable events on the horizon.

By mid-June, Margaret Nutt was still collecting Peanut and me from school at the end of the day. However, my mother did not like this situation, and within days of getting her new car she had a terrible argument with my father over the school-run.

What began with my mother telling my father that she did not want Margaret Nutt bringing me home from school any more, within moments became a screaming rage, during which my mother accused my father of having an affair with Margaret. Of course, there was no truth in the allegation. However, my mother began screaming foul obscenities. Anyone would think they had actually had sex. But I, knowing my father and the timid Margaret Nutt, knew there could be no truth in the accusation. My mother began screaming threats to go and have the matter out on Margaret Nutt's doorstep.

In the end my father managed to defuse the situation, but not before he agreed to end the school-run arrangement with Margaret Nutt. From now on, my mother declared, *she* would collect me from school. I sat on the stairs listening to this, and felt my heart sinking. I knew that my mother was once again imposing her very powerful personality on my father.

With my mother back in the house she began to taint every good thing that happened to me. I lived in perpetual fear of what she was about to do next. There were two things that were going to be factors in my mother's war against me.

My father had bought me a dog for my birthday, a Springer spaniel puppy I named Skip. Vicky was very jealous of my new pet, but not being a selfish kind of child I was quite willing to share Skip with her and Ingrid and let them play with him whenever they wanted.

The other element in this tale of disaster was that I still had incontinence problems. Since I'd had this problem all my life I had learnt a variety of coping skills, the main one being to keep going to the loo all the time to keep my bladder empty. Now, aged twelve, there was still the odd minor accident, but my condition was improving as I grew older. I was determined not to give my mother any excuse to accuse me of being infantile, and tried very hard not to have accidents.

The end of the school year at Kings brought with it my school report, and a letter from the headmaster asking my parents to visit him. My report was abysmal. My teachers rated me at the bottom of ability, not only because I'd had no education for nearly three years, but because I got so easily upset and agitated, and the teachers found this very hard to manage. The comment was made that they felt I had behavioural problems that they could not cope with. In a frank discussion with my parents the headmaster told them that despite the allowances he was prepared to make for my lack of educable skills and behavioural problems, he felt that a more productive environment for me would be outside mainstream education.

My father had hoped I would flourish back in Britain. My mother, on the other hand, came away from the meeting angry. My father had to face facts, she declared. I was a child with mental problems; my father's 'grand experiment' (as she sarcastically called it) had failed. There was no choice now other than a special school.

My father reluctantly agreed, not realising my mother's ulterior motives, which soon became clear. During June my mother had been in touch with a top private girls' school in Cardiff. However, the school was exclusive and very expensive, the fees twice what it had cost my father to send me to Kings.

My mother was determined that Vicky should have the best education available. However, my father could not afford to send both Vicky and me to private schools. I, considered a mental child prone to psychotic illness, was less important. Vicky was to get the top-flight education.

Since my return to Britain in the October of 1974, I had been allocated a social worker named Sally Martin, who had taken a keen interest in me. It was she who had suggested that I go to Kings.

Sally had also arranged for me to come under the paediatric psychiatrist at Whichurch Hospital, who issued my father with a Mental Health Certificate that classed me as disordered with mild autism and prevalence to psychosis. I would one day overturn this assessment, but this would take years to accomplish. The only condition I did have caused me to suffer from periods of psychotic illness, triggered by stress and mistreatment by my mother, but no one realised this yet.

My parents called Sally Martin, and told her about their meeting with Mr Beavan, who had declared I was unsuitable for education at Kings. The result was that Sally said she'd make arrangements to locate a place for me at a special school.

In July, my father was again contacted by the office of the Israeli Premier, Yitzhak Rabin. He was asked to fly to Tel Aviv for a briefing, then go to Damascus, before returning to Israel to report on his unofficial meeting with Syrian officials. He would be away for twelve days.

To my father's surprise my mother had no objections.

If my father wanted to go to the Middle East (for which he was being very well paid), my mother announced that he must go ahead.

I listened in astonishment at my mother being so reasonable. I could not find it within me to forgive her for what she had done to me in Greece. However, in the last weeks of July my mother had seemingly been all sweetness and light, and I slowly began to let my guard down.

It did not take long for my mother to revert to her normal behaviour. Within an hour of waving my father off, my mother was on the telephone to Sally Martin, claiming I was unstable and dangerous, and that she'd caught me hitting two-year-old Ingrid in a frenzy. It was a barefaced lie. Ingrid was quite happily playing with Vicky in the sitting room. I tried to protest and, God knows why, told my mother *I* was sorry. She spun from the phone and gave me a resounding slap across the face.

'You had better arrange something, and quick,' she declared to the social worker, 'What will you do if he seriously injures Ingrid?'

There were more bitter words exchanged, and the old phrases 'autistic', 'psychotic', 'disturbed and dangerous', were bandied about. My mother had learnt that these key words – this magical formula – always got her what she wanted.

Sally Martin promised my mother to find emergency placement for me. But it would, she warned, be difficult to

locate a respite place at such short notice for a child classified as autistic with mild psychosis, there being a very
limited number of beds in Cardiff. My mother would just
have to accept whatever was offered.

When my mother put the phone down, in tears I pleaded
with her not to send me away.

'I don't want you, and I *hate* you!' my mother declared. 'I
won't be responsible for you, so off you go!'

Later that afternoon, the same day as my father's departure, Sally Martin telephoned my mother. She had found a
place for me. It was far from ideal, not really being desig-
nated a respite unit, but it was the only child psychiatric bed
she could locate for me at such short notice. Indeed, if it had
not been for my Mental Health Certificate stating I had an
autistic disorder, even that would not have been offered.

'Yes … I understand …' my mother answered, her replies
terse and staccato. 'Okay,' she finally said. 'I'll take him there
tomorrow morning. You're sure they'll take him?'

More discussion.

I gathered from listening to this one-sided conversation
that I was to be taken to Ely Mental Hospital, which was a
ten-minute drive away in a shabby district of Cardiff.

And so it was that the following morning I found myself
bundled into an old yellow shirt and red tracksuit trousers,
and my mother produced a Woolworth's carrier bag into
which she had flung some clothes.

I didn't even get to say goodbye to my sisters. I was
roughly shoved out of the house, put into the back of her
car, and taken the short drive to Ely Hospital.

Ely Hospital was a squalid-looking Victorian redbrick complex of several big buildings. I would one day discover Ely was what was called in the sixties and seventies a 'Subnormality Hospital' for males with 'special needs' including autism, which was how Sally Martin had managed such a short-notice temporary placement for me.

My mother dragged me sobbing out of the car. History – with an evil sense of déjà vu – was repeating itself. Despite knowing that my father would be back in ten days, I was terrified.

My mother took no notice of my anguish. She dragged me into the building, my arm gripped painfully in one hand, my carrier bag of clothes in the other. She had a few brief words with a man who came out of an office to see her; she got my Mental Health certificate out of her handbag, signed some papers, and then was gone without so much as a second glance in my direction.

Very distressed and sobbing, I allowed myself to be led away by a nurse down long corridors, across a courtyard, and into a dingy-looking building. The nurse took out a key, unlocked a door, and took me on to the ward. I was shaking uncontrollably by now, and the sight of twenty mentally impaired boys in the big day room, which smelt strongly of disinfectant, did nothing to alleviate my distress. I kept telling myself, 'My father doesn't know I'm here.' The nurse took me into a big dormitory of twenty beds, and put my carrier bag into a bedside cupboard. I was then led back to the day room, where I took myself off into a corner, squatted on the floor, and sobbed my heart out.

'I should not be here,' I told myself, 'not in a place like this. I've done nothing wrong.' It had happened again; my mother had put me into a mental hospital.

All the boys were aged between nine and thirteen. Most played on the floor, but it couldn't be called normal play. They clattered, banged, and threw things, which the nurses kept picking up. The three nurses would also intervene to prevent the children becoming aggressive. The staff didn't seem to dress half the boys, who were still in their pyjamas at midday. Two of the boys were very impaired: one sat on the floor and clung to a teddy bear. Another boy, attired only in a nappy and pyjama jacket, had an infant's dummy; he just sat staring into space, completely unaware of his surroundings. At the far end of the long day room were a cluster of adolescent-sized high-chairs, wherein sat the more disturbed boys, all in their nightwear, and with table-tops and pommels affixed to prevent them getting up.

Why, I asked myself, was my life so dreadful?

I knew the answer to that: my mother hated me because I had failed my mental assessments, been classified as autistic, psychotic, and had problems with my bladder. She loved my sisters, but I don't believe she loved my father. He was a means to an end, and all she wanted from him was his support – both physical and financial – to give her doted-upon daughters the best in life.

Bedtime at Ely Hospital was early, at 7 p.m. on a bright sunny evening. After being stripped naked and taken to what was called the 'sloosh room' where the boys were made to stand against a tiled wall and washed, I found

myself put into hospital-issue terry-lined PVC incontinence pants. A nurse then bundled me unceremoniously
into the dormitory, where she opened my Woolworth's
carrier bag, only to find there were no pyjamas. Instead, to
my mortification, she produced one of my pale-green anti-
strip all-in-ones.

I became hysterical, pleading not to be put in the hated
garment, and ran into a corner of the dormitory, kicking
out when the nurse came near. In the frantic struggle I
accidentally struck her face. Of course, she lost her temper
and called for help from two nurses, who came running
across the dormitory. Between them they wrestled me to
the floor, got the all-in-one on me, and sat on me while
they did up the rubber buttons. The three of them then
picked me up off the floor and put me into my bed. I knew
to struggle was futile, so I just lay in bed and sobbed until
I fell asleep.

On the following morning a nurse undid my all-in-one,
and I was allowed to get dressed. I had my breakfast and
returned to my corner of the day room, to sit and stare at
the mentally disordered boys.

By lunchtime, I was becoming progressively more and
more agitated and distressed at my predicament. I wasn't
mentally deranged. I should not be here, my mind screamed,
not in this place of mental children. I wanted to be at home
with my dad.

I could tell I was deteriorating because I had begun to
hear my mother shouting hateful things at me; my mind
was playing evil tricks. I knew I was becoming mentally ill

again, and very quickly. I had to get out of this place, and soon if I was not to become psychotic again. I became paranoid – deluded – convinced that my mother had now succeeded in getting rid of me, and these nurses were colluding with her, willing accomplices to lock me away from my dad.

Suddenly I snapped, and ran across the day room to the main door, screaming to be let out, kicking and hitting the locked ward door in a frenzy. Two nurses pounced on me, and held me flat on the floor until I calmed down, but I would not. I screamed hysterically, beating my head savagely up and down on the polished floor.

A male nurse was called, and between the three of them they held me still to stop me hurting myself. As I lay held face down on the floor, I watched a nurse come over, syringe in hand. My sleeve was rolled up, my flesh pinched, and they injected me. Within a minute or two all my resistance was gone, and I became disorientated and floppy. The nurses picked me up off the floor, and sat me in an easy chair. I was just staring vacantly into space by now, feeling very tired, my state of awareness impaired.

The nurses at Ely Hospital kept me sedated and in my all-in-one for the next three days for misbehaving and exhibiting gross disturbance; this treatment every day made me easier to manage.

Then, one day, on getting up the nurse produced my clothes and allowed me to get dressed in T-shirt and track-suit trousers.

I was then taken into the day room, placed standing in a huddle with eight other dressed boys waiting by the locked ward door. Several nurses then took us off the ward, and through a doorway into an outside yard. I use the word 'yard' loosely, for it was actually a tarmaced area abutting the children's building, divided into a series of runs, like rats' cages made of ten-foot-high chain-linked fence and a series of locked gates. We were divided into two groups of four boys. Each group was then put in a separate locked 'run'. It was very humiliating because the runs were visible from the main access road within Ely Hospital, and nurses, passers-by, and visitors, all stared at us as we milled about, or clung to the fence looking out.

We were left outside all morning until brought in for lunch, after which we spent the rest of the afternoon on the ward. The same procedure was adopted for the next four days. There was nothing to do; the boys didn't even talk or play with each other. There was one sole activity conducted as if by consensus. We all stood at the end of the runs, and watched in silence as people went by.

Eventually my ordeal ended one day when a nurse produced my Woolworth's carrier bag and took me off the ward. She took me back to the main building, where my mother stood waiting, and we left for home.

It was a curious journey home, for what should have taken ten minutes took closer to thirty as my mother began to drive aimlessly about the suburbs, then out into the countryside. Eventually she deigned to speak.

'It'll be no good you crying to Dad, you know,' she said at last, glancing over her shoulder to give me a glare as I sat in the back.

She returned her concentration to the road for a moment.

'He's mine now,' she stated, as if I were in a contest with her. 'You don't matter. If you don't want to be sent back to that place for good then you'll say nothing.'

I didn't reply.

'I can do it, do it all!' she suddenly screamed at me over her shoulder. 'If you get in my way, I'll get rid of you for good!'

I began to cry, shattered by my ordeal at Ely Hospital, terrified of my mother. She stopped the car in a farm gateway, and turned to look at me huddled in the corner on the back seat.

'Promise me ...' she said in a sing-song voice, far more terrifying than a shout. Her eyes gazed at me from behind her spectacles, cold and hard as obsidian and just as soulless. 'Promise me ... or back you go ... back you go right now ...'

Terrified, I nodded my head and promised her my fidelity. It felt as if I was selling my soul ...

My father returned home the following day, and to my astonishment my mother quite openly told him she'd sent me to Ely Hospital for a week's respite.

He asked me how it had been, to which I replied that I didn't want to go back there. I even pleaded with him to leave me with my grandmother the next time he went away.

Over his shoulder I saw my mother shoot me an evil glance, her mouth open in preparation to say something.

However, before she could interrupt, my father shook his head.

'No,' he said, 'because of your mental problems and your grandmother's age, it's not possible.'

My mother smirked at me over my father's shoulder. She had won again. She would always win against me.

CHAPTER 11

A Decline Destined to Happen

During August of 1975 my parents had some terrible arguments over Vicky and me. My father wanted to persevere with private education for me, but he was faced with the undeniable fact that I had failed at Kings. Under persistent pressure from my mother, day in, day out, my father's resolve began to weaken. Finally, he telephoned Sally Martin, and told her to set the wheels in motion to send me to Meadowbank Special School.

My father felt utterly defeated by the end of August 1975. However, he should have listened to his conscience, which told him this was wrong. His first mistake was to have taken my mother back. But he was yet to realise that in the summer of 1975, yet to realise the evil he had let into his house …

At the beginning of September, Vicky was kitted out to attend her new school with skirt and blazer, straw boater, white knee socks and patent-leather shoes. My mother was ecstatic that her long-term plans for Vicky were coming to fruition.

I, on the other hand, lived at the opposite extremity of existence. There was no uniform requirement at Meadowbank School. All the children had mental problems. In my class of fifteen, four were mildly autistic, and the rest seemed to my eyes manic and threw things all the time. Education at Meadowbank was limited to a little reading and writing, the emphasis being on art every afternoon.

However, at this stage, all was strangely calm. It wasn't until November, when my father was asked by the Israelis to go to Cairo for diplomatic talks with the Egyptian government, that things became extremely bad for me.

When my father told my mother that he had been asked to go to Cairo, she seemed happy for him to go. Everything was going her way. She had plenty of money, a nice house and a new car. She encouraged him, saying she would manage quite well on her own.

The day of my father's departure came, and off he went with a smile on his face, blissfully ignorant that his wife was an unstable psychopath. As soon as my father had driven away my mother closed the front door and pulled me to one side while Vicky took Ingrid by the hand and led her to the sitting room.

'You're not going to play me up, are you?' my mother demanded, her eyes flashing dangerously.

Terrified of her, I shook my head.

My mother seemed content to leave it at that, and let go of me to head down the hall to the kitchen.

Carl Gustav Jung, the Swiss philosopher and psychiatrist, was the creator of a theory he named 'synchronicity'.

Synchronicity is the coming together of coincidences – people, current affairs, chance encounters, and random events – that can result in a particular though unpredictable outcome. Such an act of Jung's synchronicity was about to take place that day, sending me off into a life-changing direction, and nothing would ever be the same again.

The day my father left for Israel – Saturday, 20 November 1975 – proceeded just like any other. It was a wet November weekend, so I passed the time playing with Skip and Ingrid, who in her toddlerish way adored my young dog.

About mid-afternoon the doorbell rang.

Vicky went to answer the door, and moments later I heard her call our mother. I caught a fleeting glance of her as she headed down the hall.

I didn't think much of it until I heard a wail of anguish emanate from my mother, and much urgent conversation. Puzzled, I left Ingrid and went out to the hall and saw my mother talking to a policeman.

I could tell that something serious had happened, because my mother was almost hysterical. A policewoman appeared in the hall, and led my mother into the drawing room.

'What's going on?' I asked Vicky.

'It's Dad,' she said. 'He's had a bad accident in the car.'

I began to tremble, a sign of an oncoming anxiety attack.

'It's okay, sonny,' the policeman said. 'Your dad's going to be fine.'

His words didn't penetrate. I began shaking and thought that I was going to faint.

'Here,' said the policeman to Vicky, her height giving her a maturity beyond her years. 'Is he all right?'

'No. He's a bit mental,' Vicky responded. 'I'll see to him. Just look after my mum, please.' And she pushed me towards the staircase.

By the time Vicky had pushed me up the stairs, I was having a full-blown panic attack.

As I trembled and shook, she bundled me into my room, and before I realised what she was doing, closed the door and turned the key in the lock. She actually had the temerity to lock me in my room out of the way until the crisis was resolved.

Despite my anxiety attack, I was furious with her.

I was left in my room until teatime, by which time the details of my father's accident had become known. My mother had even spoken to him on the telephone.

My father's car had collided with a lorry on the motorway near Reading. The car was a write-off, his injuries severe. He had a broken arm and collarbone, torn shoulder ligaments, cuts, grazes, and concussion, but his life was not in danger. He was in Reading Hospital, where he would stay for about ten days, before my mother could go and collect him.

On Monday morning my mother telephoned Sally Martin. She told her of our family crisis, that my father had been badly injured. She claimed that she couldn't cope with me on her own, that I was aggressive towards Ingrid and unstable, and requested an emergency respite admission for me to Ely Hospital until she could sort things out. Having already been in Ely Hospital that summer seemed to make a repeat admission for me easier. Sally telephoned back within an hour to tell my mother there was a bed available and she could take me in any time that day.

At first I didn't know what was happening, for my mother didn't tell me what she had done. She just went upstairs and began to throw a few items of my clothing into a carrier bag. I asked my mother what was going on. It was a question that received a disproportionately aggressive response.

She threw me against the bedroom wall, and began screaming at me insanely, her spittle landing all over my face.

'I can't stand you,' she screamed. 'I *hate* you! Your dad's hurt and I've got your sisters to consider. I don't want you, do you hear! You're going back to Ely right now!'

At the sudden realisation of what was going to happen, that I was being sent to Ely Hospital, I dropped to the floor, threw my arms around her legs, and pleaded not to be sent away.

'I won't go!' I wailed. 'I'll run away. I'll go to Nan's. She won't let you send me there!'

I had challenged my mother head on, a fatal mistake.

Yanking me to my feet, she threw me against the wardrobe with a resounding bang.

'You will go,' she snarled, her face an inch from mine. 'If you play me up, I'll kill Skip!'

My blood ran cold at the words of horror erupting from her lips, at the expression of hate on her face. All my resistance evaporated, and I fell to the floor in tears. My mother stood over me, triumphant and knowing she would use the ultimate terror weapon if I resisted in any way.

Twenty minutes later I was bundled out of the house, shoved into the back of her car, and taken the short drive to Ely Hospital.

Placed back on the same ward of mentally disordered boys, I withdrew into myself. I just sat on the floor in the corner, had a good cry, and refused to have anything to do with anyone.

To my utter mortification, on the first evening there I found that my mother had again not packed me any pyjamas, and all I had to wear were the horrible all-in-ones.

Determined that my father should rescue me and throw my mother out of the house for doing this to me, I played up dreadfully from the first moment of my arrival. I refused to cooperate in any way. I refused to eat; refused to sit when told to; I sobbed for hours every day to go home; I placed myself by the locked ward door all day long, looking for an opportunity to run away.

I came to be considered a problem case, a disturbed autistic child with psychosis. The consequence was that the staff retaliated by leaving me in just my all-in-one twenty-four hours a day, every day, because it made me easier to manage.

After a few days of being very difficult, becoming frantic when I beat my head on the walls and floor, hammering my fists on the locked ward door, screaming to be let out, the staff suddenly lost all patience with me one morning when

I lashed out at a nurse who was trying to get me away from the door. My first inkling that something bad was about to happen was when two nurses and a male nurse grabbed me, and wrestled me to the floor. Before I knew what was happening, as I screamed and sobbed to them to leave me alone, they picked me up off the floor and carried me kicking and screaming across the day room to the high-chairs. It took all three nurses to hold me down, to affix the pommel and table-top so I could not get up. Then, while I struggled and screamed, the two women held my arms until the male nurse rolled up my sleeve, grabbed a handful of arm, and injected me with a strong sedative. From now on that was where I stayed every day, from getting up at 8 a.m. until bedtime at 7 p.m., when two nurses would strip and shower me. Because of my diagnosed autism and prevalence to psychosis, the practitioner at Ely increased my dose of the tranquillising anti-psychotic Chlorpromazine, and I was also given Valium every day to keep me quiet.

It was under these circumstances that I was kept at Ely for three weeks, and I began to rapidly deteriorate mentally. I alternated between sedated zombification, and being completely psychotic when I could hear voices talking and shouting at me. I would sob and scream my head off, but the nurses had decided I was a troublesome psychotic autistic child, and I was kept seated from now on with the six other disturbed boys in the high-chairs.

Kept sedated all day to keep me quiet, I was one day dozing in my high-chair when I heard a familiar voice calling my name …

'Alex … Alex … Alex …'

I opened my eyes and, heavily sedated as I was, beheld my father standing in front of me.

My father looked aghast at my predicament, and kept glancing around the room at the very mental children I was living with. He had never seen anything like it before.

My previous hospital admission to St Lawrence's Hospital had been to a psychiatric unit, and even then we'd met in the quiet stability of a visitors' room. I noticed his jacket was draped over his shoulders, concealing his arm in a sling. My father bent down to peer into my face.

The nurse was talking to my parents, but I could only pick up snippets of what was being said: 'He's very psychotic … He's been self-harming, so he needs to be kept securely seated … he's delusional too … keeps saying his mother wants to kill him … He lives completely in a world of his own … He keeps asking for a friend called Skip, who he says is dead …'

At that statement my father snapped upright, and gave the nurse a hard look. Then his words entered my head and seared into my brain for ever: 'Skip's not a person,' he said. 'It's his dog who died the day he came here …'

My father got no further, for I began to cry, desperate to be out of the seat, and all the while screaming, 'Oh, Skip's dead … Skip's dead …'

Everything seemed to happen in slow motion. The nurse rushed over to hold my arms down to stop me hurting myself, and she was shouting something. Another nurse rushed over, rolled my sleeve up, jabbed a little needle into my arm and injected me; then they pinned my arms down until the drug gained the upper hand, and all the while I mumbled over and over again 'Skip … Skip … Skip …'

My mother told my father that Skip had got out of the back garden and had been run over. However, many years later my belief that my mother had killed Skip was confirmed when Vicky told me that Mother had given him a massive overdose of paracetamol and Valium in his food, and he died the first night I was at Ely Hospital.

Following my parents' visit to me that day in mid-December, I became very depressed and mentally ill. After my father met with the unit practitioner, the nurses eased up on me. The practice of putting me in the high-chair ceased, although I was kept in the all-in-one. I was no longer a nuisance, did not hang around the ward door looking for the opportunity to run away. What was the point? My father hadn't taken me home. I spent all my time mourning the loss of Skip. Despite what my mother had told my father I knew she had done it. She had really killed my puppy; it was so monstrous it was beyond my comprehension.

I didn't scream or even beat my head on the floor in anguish anymore. What was the point? Skip was dead, just like Nikki in Greece. Now I had two deaths on my conscience. Despite everything that the doctors had told me in Germany I was still convinced that Nikki's death was my fault. Now my mother had killed Skip because of me. Just like a pebble tossed down a cliff can cause an avalanche, I began to go downhill mentally.

I was in Ely Hospital for another week after my parents came to see me. My father was very angry that my mother had sent me there, particularly because he knew how traumatic it had been for me in the mental asylum in Greece. All my progress and cure had been undone in a few brief weeks. That I remained at Ely another week was due largely to my mental condition. In my case it had been easier for my mother to get me *into* Ely, than it was for my father to get me *out* again.

I was eventually discharged from Ely Hospital a week before Christmas, but by then I had suffered a complete psychotic collapse. The day after coming home, Father took me to see my psychiatrist at Whichurch Hospital. Dr Evans was concerned by my decline, and told my father that the place for me had *not* been Ely Hospital. Ely was a hospital for mentally handicapped children and adults. Dr Evans was incredibly frustrated because by late 1975 he had concluded my mental problems were primarily psychotic in nature, and probably not mild autism at all. Dr Evans appreciated I had been assessed as mildly autistic when I was eight, but he was becoming convinced this was a mistaken diagnosis.

After talking to me, during which I kept insisting my mother hated me, that she had killed my dog, that she would kill me too, that I could hear my mother and a man's 'voice' talking to me, Dr Evans was of the opinion that I was completely psychotic again.

Dr Evans told my father to take me home for Christmas. It would be necessary to admit me to a psychiatric hospital in January, but that was going to be extremely difficult because there were very few child psychiatric beds in South Wales.

Over Christmas I just sat in the sitting room in a daze, not really taking anything in because I completely lost touch with reality. I withdrew into my own closed-in world, one in which the 'voice' and my mother took turns to shout and taunt me, and I was completely unable to stop them.

My mum had killed Skip. She had actually done it. That meant she could do anything, break any law, do whatever she wanted, and I was terrified of her. I didn't dare speak. I mustn't move. I must stay in my chair, or stand in the corner, or sit at the table. I must just do whatever she wanted or she would kill me too, and my father would be powerless to stop her.

A few days into January, Sally Martin came out to the house to see me. I sat in pyjamas and dressing gown in the sitting room, staring vacantly into space. I knew Sally was there, and I can remember her kneeling before me, holding my face in both her cool hands and saying: 'Hello, sweet pea. How are you?'

I didn't dare move. I just stared through her at my mother standing behind her.

'Be careful,' said the sing-song melodic 'voice' in my head. 'If you move or say anything, I'll kill you ...'

Two large tears erupted from my eyes and ran down my face.

My parents and Sally had a long conversation, but I wasn't listening to anyone any more. The only voice I took notice of was the man's 'voice' that threatened to hurt me if I so much as moved my hands out of my lap.

Major decisions had been taken for me, and Sally had come to tell my parents that a bed on a children's psychiatric ward had become available. There was only one drawback, she said, and that was that it was quite distant, on the other side of Abergavenny, some 50 miles away, at a big psychiatric hospital called Pen-y-Fal, in the Monmouthshire countryside.

The following afternoon, Ingrid and Vicky having been left with my grandmother, Dad, Mum and I set off for Abergavenny. We travelled in my father's new Mark III Ford Cortina, my mother driving because Dad's arm was still in a sling.

I had been given a lot of Valium before we left the house to keep me quiet during the long journey. It was a cold afternoon, so Mother had produced my new anorak to keep me warm. She had impatiently pulled it on me, hood up, and yanked the zip all the way up under my chin.

So there I sat, disorientated, sedated, and bundled up, gazing out of the window as we headed up the Welsh Valleys, through Treforest and Merthyr Tydfil. Eventually, the drab terraced housing of the valleys gave way to wild countryside bordering the Heads of the Valley Road. All the traffic had headlights on by the time we arrived at the market town of Abergavenny, the rain beginning to turn to wet sleet.

It was at this point that I was suddenly sick in the back of Dad's new car, over the upholstery, carpet, and my new anorak. There was angry shouting by my mother as she drove, but we were almost at our destination, Neville Hall General Hospital on the outskirts of Abergavenny. I just sat cocooned in my anorak, sobbing to myself.

Mum soon turned in through the entrance into a vast modern complex that was Neville Hall. She drove between the buildings until we came to a car park before a Victorian building at the back of the main complex.

The purpose for coming here was that the psychiatrist from Pen-y-Fal Hospital had decided to conduct my admission at Neville Hall, not at the secluded Pen-y-Fal Hospital out on the Monmouth Road. It was by now late on a winter's afternoon.

My mother parked the car, and yanked me out of the back to assess the damage. I was pinned between two cars, Dad holding my arm. Mum went to the boot, took out a towel, and proceeded to wipe the anorak clean. After several minutes rubbing, she yanked the hood and zip down, and pulled the coat off me and threw it in the boot. The cold air on my back, the sleet on my neck and hands felt like small electric shocks.

I began to cry again because I felt so awful. I was cold, sick, and terrified by my surroundings, the garish yellow glow from the streetlights turning everything shades of grey.

A minibus entered the car park and parked in the corner. The driver stayed seated, but a suited man and a nurse in a cape with a bag in hand got out, and gave me a long stare as they walked past.

Eventually my mother finished cleaning the car. She produced my holdall from the boot, held my arm, Dad on the other side, and we set off across the car park to the forbidding-looking building.

By now I was freezing cold and very distressed. Halfway across the car park I refused to go on. My mother handed the holdall to my father, grabbed me by both shoulders, and shook and shook me. I let my legs collapse under me to fall on to my bottom in the wet, sobbing and refusing to go on. My mother lost her temper. She grabbed me by my armpits. When she picked me up I was astonished by her strength. She began to lay into me, slapping my cold wet legs as hard as she could.

'Oh, for heaven's sake, Voula ...' my father began.

'Shut up,' my mother snapped. 'I won't have him playing up.'

'Move or I'll hurt you ...' the sing-song voice erupted in my head.

My eyes opened wide in terror. *He* was here. *He* was watching me. *He* and my mother were in cahoots.

My mother dug hard fingers into my arm, and I allowed myself to be hustled up the steps into the Victorian building.

The door slammed shut behind us with a resounding bang. The foyer was deserted, but immediately a tall thin man with curly hair stuck his head out of a door, and told my parents he was the psychiatrist supervising my case at Pen-y-Fal Hospital.

He led the way into an office, a bare consulting room

with four chairs and a desk. I was pushed to sit on the chair in the middle of the room, my parents taking the two seats on one side. A nurse in her cape sat behind the desk. The psychiatrist perched on a corner of the desk, and sat staring at me for a long moment.

Eventually he said something to the nurse, who opened a file on the desk, and turned it around for him to read. He spent some moments reading, flicking back to check something, then returned to the page he had been studying.

He began to talk to my parents about me as I sat terrified, staring at my hands in my lap. All the old key phrases were spoken between my parents and the psychiatrist during their conversation: 'abnormal behaviour', 'psychosis', 'hears voices', 'delusional', 'has tantrums'.

He asked when I'd first exhibited the symptoms of psychotic delusions and disorder. My mother told the doctor she believed I had always had it, certainly since the age of six or seven; it had just taken until I was eight to get a diagnosis.

The psychiatrist nodded. The question he proposed to my parents was how serious was the condition. Was this an acute psychotic episode? Or could it be the beginnings of schizophrenia?

At this my father intervened, pointing out that I'd had periods of remission. Was that not a hopeful sign? he asked, desperate for any words of hope.

'That remains to be seen, doesn't it?' the psychiatrist responded. 'We can treat him at Pen-y-Fal, but a lot is going to be up to Alexander.'

I stared at my lap. I was cold, wet, and very frightened, because the people in the room were not the only voices I could hear. The 'voice' kept threatening me, kept telling me 'we' will get you. I didn't know who 'we' were. I concluded in my confused way that 'we' was the hospital I was being sent to. That terrified me more than anything else, and I had a knot of fear deep in my stomach.

'Alexander!'

I suddenly realised that the psychiatrist was talking to me, had been calling me for some moments. Why hadn't I heard him?

'Alexander!' someone else shouted from behind me. I jumped and turned around to see who else was in the room. There was no one there.

'Alex!'

I jerked back to face the psychiatrist.

'Did you hear someone?' he asked. 'Is there someone else in this room?'

Wide-eyed and terrified, I nodded my head.

The psychiatrist pursed his lips.

'Who is it?' he asked.

'I don't know,' I sobbed. 'It's *him* and he won't leave me alone.'

'Where is he?'

'I don't know …' I wailed. 'Sometimes he talks from the television. But today I don't know where he is.'

'He can't hurt you, you know,' the psychiatrist told me.

'He can,' I insisted. 'Sometimes he grabs my hands or arms …'

The psychiatrist looked at the nurse. 'Delusional with tactile hallucinations,' he said, and she wrote it down in my file.

'Do you know why you're here?' he asked me.

'Yes. My mum hates me.' I decided to spill the beans, my final plea to get my father to see she was a malignant force out to get rid of me.

'She hates me,' I repeated. 'She tried to kill me in Greece. She killed my dog. Now she's threatened to hurt me – to kill me – if I get in her way.'

My mother blew through her lips in a hoot of derision.

'You can see what I'm up against,' she told the doctor. 'He's completely crazy. There's nothing I can do with him, and I'm afraid to leave him alone with his infant sister. I think he's dangerous.'

'Got you,' the 'voice' behind me shouted. 'Now you'll go away for ever …'

I glanced behind me again, sure there was someone there.

'Has someone spoken to you again, Alex?' the psychiatrist asked.

I nodded, wringing my hands anxiously in my lap.

The psychiatrist transferred his attention back to my parents.

'You'll have to leave him with us. I think he's very mentally ill.'

'How long will it last?' asked my father.

'I think you'd better forget him and get on with your lives, at least in the short term,' the psychiatrist said with

231

some finality. 'He's completely psychotic, and it may take a long time before we see any improvement ...'

'He's recovered in the past,' my father responded, desperate for the slightest hope to cling on to.

The psychiatrist nodded. 'Yes, he'll probably recover, but I think it's going to take a long time. On the basis of my examination of him, and his notes sent up by Dr Evans, I'm going to section him. That means I'm going to detain him under the Mental Health Act for three months.'

'Detain him for three months ...' my father echoed, aghast.

'Yes,' the psychiatrist replied. 'It's just a formality that will allow us to take all his care decisions, decide what medication and treatment we need to give him. It's a legal way to transfer custody of him as a minor to us until April. We can then take a further decision to re-section, or discharge him if he's recovered.'

I just sat, feeling very small and cold, staring from face to face as the adults talked about me, petrified my father was going to leave me here.

'You're going to stay here for ever and ever ...' the 'voice' sang in my ear. 'She's got your dad now, and they'll never come back for you ...'

I let out a scream of panic, and threw myself at my father's legs and clung to him.

'Don't leave me here!' I cried. 'Mum hates me. She killed Skip, and now she's getting rid of me too!'

'Now, Alex,' my father said softly, stroking my head, 'you know that's not true.'

'It is! It is!' I cried. This was my last chance, I knew, to get him to defend me. 'She hurt me in Greece. Now she's threatened to kill me if I get in her way!' I began to sob hysterically.

'This is getting us nowhere,' the psychiatrist said. 'I'm going to admit him now, and we'll take him to Pen-y-Fal.'

'Yes,' my father agreed. 'What happens now?'

'Well, I've brought the paperwork. Dr Evans at Whichurch Hospital has already signed the section order; it just needs my counter-signature to validate the order.'

'No! No! No!' I shrieked, scrambling up off the floor to try to stop the psychiatrist signing the paperwork.

My father put an arm around my waist and held me as I struggled. I watched in horror as the psychiatrist produced a pen and began to fill in the form, eventually signing it with a flourish.

'Ha, ha,' said the 'voice' in a sudden shout. 'Now you're never going home, ever, ever again …'

I began to scream. I let my legs buckle under me and fell to the floor, beating my head upon the linoleum in frustration, only to be firmly grasped by my father and the psychiatrist, put up on to my chair and held there.

The 'voice' was shouting at me all through this, taunting rambling nonsense, and I could not concentrate on what was being said.

The psychiatrist was talking to the nurse, who reached into her bag to produce a slim black case. I screamed in anguish and struggled to be free of both my father and doctor as she opened the case on the desk and produced and syringe and needle, and a small glass bottle.

'Ten mils please,' the psychiatrist said.

The syringe was filled from the bottle, and a little squirt of fluid was ejected from the needle.

Mum and Dad held me. The nurse handed the syringe to the psychiatrist and then rolled my sleeve up. The psychiatrist bent over me, but I screamed and pulled away. He grasped my upper arm and stuck the needle into me.

Everyone stayed holding me for a few minutes, until the tension in my limbs subsided, and I became all floppy and sleepy.

One of the last things I can remember from that traumatic day was the psychiatrist saying, 'I think it's time we went, don't you Alex?'

I didn't reply. I buried my face in my father's arms, taking in the comforting smell of him, and wouldn't move. Hands grasped me, and pulled me off my father. I wanted to cry, but I was all cried out and too sleepy. My mum handed my holdall to the psychiatrist, and we left the office.

It was snowing outside, cold wet snow that didn't settle. My father gave me a hug, then helped lift me up into the back of the minibus. There were a few more words said, but I was too sleepy to care. I flopped on the seat, my face pressed against the cold glass, and the nurse sat next to me. The psychiatrist got in next to the driver, and it began to pull away.

I watched out of the window as Mum and Dad stood in the falling snow. My father waved to me; I did not wave back. My eyes felt funny; I was so sleepy, and my face was wet and clammy from tears I could not stop.

CHAPTER 12

Psychotic at Pen-y-Fal

I lay in bed and stared around my Spartan room, which contained a bed, chair, and bedside cupboard. My gaze settled on the window. Outside it was raining, and large raindrops from a winter squall ran down the glass.

I'd spent most of yesterday at the window staring at the outside world; my only view was the rear car park and the countryside beyond. I knew there would be nothing new to see this morning.

This was my fourth day at Pen-y-Fal. Or was it still only my third? I had lost track of time already and wondered whether it was Thursday or Friday. When I had seen the psychiatrist yesterday he'd asked me what day it was. I didn't know, and he found that significant, noting my ignorance in my file.

I hated that file, with its claims that I was delusional, psychotic, and hated my mother, who in reality hated me; she was determined to be rid of me and had killed my dog. It was that file that determined my place in the world, for within the buff folder were papers that declared me psychotic and not allowed out of hospital until the psychiatrist decided I was 'cured'.

On my arrival at Pen-y-Fal that first evening I had been extremely distressed and in a state of complete mental collapse. I could hear the 'voice' taunting me as if he knew my every thought before it sprang into my mind. I had lain on my bed sobbing uncontrollably for hours, frantically screaming to shut up the 'voice', and in the end they gave me an injection and I fell asleep.

The following morning a nurse had come into my room with a smile as I stood in my pyjamas staring out of the window. After giving me tablets and a sweet pink syrup that was evidently some form of medication, she had produced my dressing gown and slippers, and taken me to see the ward.

As we walked down the corridor I was told this was Ward 3, a boys' ward for ages ten to sixteen. Although I was in a single room at the moment, the nurse said this was only until I had been stabilised. Once I'd settled in I would be moved to one of the three dormitories that had six beds. She had opened a door and showed me a pleasant room with six beds, posters of cars and planes on the walls.

Continuing down the corridor I had been shown a very big day room, with easy chairs, a television, several bookshelves at one end, two dining tables at the far end. I eyed the television warily; the 'voice' had often emanated from the television at home, and I had become frightened of it.

At this point I had begun to get upset and tearful. The nurse tried to cheer me up.

'This isn't such a bad place,' she had said. 'Now I don't want any tears.'

I had nodded and tried to smile. The more normal I behaved, I told myself, the sooner they'd let me go home. But go home to what? My mother? It wouldn't just be home to my dad. There was nowhere safe for me. I began to weep at my predicament: mental hospital or my mother. The nurse didn't understand the cause of my distress, and keen not to upset the ambience of calm in the day room she ushered me back through the double-doors into the main corridor.

The young woman, who told me her name was Nurse Harris, took me to the far end of the long corridor, where she pointed to two white doors that had small windows set within them.

'These are what we call the "time-out rooms",' she said. 'If anyone becomes too difficult or aggressive, they have to do "time out" for a little while.' She gave a slightly embarrassed cough. 'You don't want to do "time out", Alex, it's not very nice. So try to be a good boy and stay nice and calm.'

She pointed to a closed door at the end of the corridor. 'This is a locked ward,' she told me, 'but you can go wherever you like on the ward. The toilets and bathrooms are down that corridor there.' She pointed down a passageway to the right.

I was still staring at the white 'time-out' doors. During my time at St Lawrence's Hospital they'd called them 'quiet rooms'. In the Greek asylum it had been an isolation cell. I knew exactly what these rooms were, whatever they were called. I forced an uncertain smile at the nurse.

'I think it's time you went back to your room,' she had said. 'The doctor will be along in a while. You'll have to spend a few days in your room, but every day you can spend a little longer in the day room, so long as you're okay and the doctor approves it.' And with that we went back to my room.

'I'll be back in a little while to see you again and bring you some books. Do you like Tintin and Asterix?' she asked.

I nodded.

She smiled and left, closing the door behind her.

At this point, having held on to myself rather unsuccessfully, I broke down and wept and wept.

All this, my first encounter with Ward 3, had been three or four days ago, and already I had lost track of time.

My door opened, and the senior nurse, Nurse Johnson, came in.

'Still in bed, Alex?' she asked. 'It's ten o'clock you know. I think it's time you got up, don't you? Come on,' she continued, 'you can spend the morning in the day room.'

I was feeling very lethargic because I'd had a bad night. Despite the medication I had awoken several times and sobbed to myself in the dark.

'What day is it?' I asked.

'Saturday,' said Nurse Johnson. 'Come on. I'll help you dress.'

She rummaged in my cupboard and got out a jumper and tracksuit trousers.

As I entered the day room Nurse Johnson propelled me towards the television, where most of the boys had gathered to watch Saturday-morning TV. There was some manic children's programme on with adults flinging custard pies and buckets of water at each other. I intensely disliked the shouting and laughter. Not keen on the television, I pulled back.

'No, Alex,' Nurse Johnson said firmly. 'I want you to sit with the others for a change, not by yourself. That's not being very friendly.'

I allowed myself to be pushed into a chair next to a boy who gave me a brief glance before turning his attention back to the television.

I suppose I had been sitting, getting increasingly disturbed by the screaming and laughter on the television for about twenty minutes, when I suddenly began to feel very disorientated by the frantic action. I slipped out of my seat to kneel on the floor.

'What are you doing?' my mother's voice suddenly asked me. 'Get up this instant, Alex. Do you hear me? Get up!'

My eyes opened wide in terror, and I found myself glancing around the room.

'Get up Alex, or I'll hurt you,' my mother warned, her silky voice both honey and poison at the same time. 'You know I'll do it! No one can stop me …'

I began to cry, and banged my head hard on the floor, desperate to stop my mother's voice.

'Get up!' my mother snapped. 'Do you hear me? Get up!'

239

I glanced at the television, a blur of movement on the screen and lots of manic adult laughter, all blended into a disorganised kaleidoscope of colour and intrusive noise.

I suddenly realised where my mother was. Her voice was coming *from* the television.

'We're coming to get you ...' said the sing-song 'voice', and he laughed.

I frantically backed away from the television, putting distance between me and it. I grasped the first thing to hand – a mug of tea on the floor next to a nurse who was sitting with the boys to watch the television. Before she could stop me, I threw her mug at the television.

It hit the screen with a bang, and smashed, sending tea everywhere. Yet still the television worked, still the laughter and manic shouting continued.

I evaded the grasp of the nurse to run away down the far end of the day room, where I hid behind the dining tables.

Suddenly there seemed to be a lot of nurses in the day room. One ushered the boys into the opposite corner; the television was switched off, and now there was no sound except my sobs of terror.

'Skip's dead and you'll be next!' my mother shouted.

I became frantic. I picked up a dining chair and threw it at the approaching nurses.

Two male nurses appeared at the run through the door, and before I could react they charged across the room.

I was sobbing hysterically by now.

'I'm sorry ... I'm sorry ...' I cried. 'Oh God, please help

me. Please make her stop shouting at me! Make her stop! Make her stop!'

The nurses glanced at each other, not knowing what I was talking about, then pounced on me. I was wrestled to the floor, and firmly held face down. And all the while I screamed at the top of my lungs.

The nurses yanked my trousers down around my knees, as I struggled against them. I felt my buttock firmly grasped, and then a sharp prick as a needle was stabbed into me, injecting me with a powerful sedative. I lay on the floor as the nurses held me down. I could still hear my mother's laughter, but my need to scream seemed to have evaporated.

Eventually I was picked up off the floor, and was briskly hustled out of the day room down the long corridor.

I was very disorientated by now, but still aware enough to notice that we passed the door to my room and kept on going down the corridor. A nurse ran ahead to open the white door to a 'time-out' room. I sobbed at them to leave me alone, but they weren't listening to me.

Many hands grabbed me and manhandled me into a white tiled room that had no window. Then my clothes were pulled off me.

Stripping me down to my pants, a nurse picked up a folded garment off the floor near the door, a white knee-length short-sleeved cotton gown, which two nurses pulled on me over my head. Then I was firmly sat on the floor; all four nurses backed out of the room, taking my clothes with them, and the door was slammed shut with a bang. A face appeared at the little window to check I remained on the floor. Then she was gone and I was all alone.

'I told you I could get you!' my mother shouted at me. 'I'm going to come and hurt you now ...' and her laughter echoed around and around.

'Sit still; don't stand; only move when I tell you ...' commanded the 'voice'.

I crawled across the floor of the small room, curled up in the corner and sobbed my heart out, and all the while my mother's hysterical laughter echoed in my head.

'I said I'd get you,' she sang at me. 'There is nowhere you can go I can't get you ...' And she went on and on.

For the rest of that day a nurse's face frequently appeared at the window to see what I was doing. I just stayed curled up in the corner, too terrified to move.

After what seemed like an eternity the door was opened, and the psychiatrist and a nurse came in; they talked to each other, but not to me. The psychiatrist did a cursory check on me, looked into my eyes, and then, while the nurse held me, gave me an injection. I remained seated on the floor, bare-legged and cold, the only overwhelming impression the stark white tiled walls and floor, the bright white light, me in a white gown. Under the influence of the drug everything began to merge into one great white miasma, a landscape of snow, and cold ice creeping up my legs and arms.

Eventually, after a very long time in 'time out' two nurses came in. They looked into my eyes, but by now I was just staring into space, disorientated and mentally isolated. Exhausted by the hours of shouting in my head.

Even my tears had dried up as my well of woe had emptied.

'Come on, Alex,' said the nurse. 'I think you can go back to your room now.'

As if in a trance, a traumatised catatonia, I allowed the two nurses to pick me up off the floor and, with legs numb and feet stumbling, walked uncertainly back down the corridor to my room.

It was dark in my room, and so they switched the light on while they got me into bed. I was given the pink syrup to drink and then some tablets. Then they left, closed my door and locked it.

The drugs soon began to take effect, and I could feel myself slipping away into sleep, and all the while was that faint voice: 'Alex … Alex … Alex …' sang my mother sweetly and mellifluously. But I was not deceived. She would kill me if she could, and I was not safe even here.

The staff learnt an important lesson that Saturday in January, when I 'flipped' and tried to smash the television. While I had been in 'time out' they had come into my room and taken away my clothes, holdall, and shoes, and I was left with just the white gown, dressing gown, and slippers. During the week that followed I was given pink syrup three times a day, and a large number of tablets that kept me sedated and calm.

I now spent all my time locked in my room, and would spend my whole day flopped on my bed, or standing at the window.

On several occasions the nurses found me screaming and

beating my head against the walls or floor, frantically hammering my fists on my door to get away from the 'voice'. The consequence was a swiftly administered injection to sedate me, and I was put to bed.

Far from recovering I was slowly declining.

One day I became very disturbed, and actually saw my mother coming out of the wall. Frantically, I began throwing the bedside cupboard and chair about my room, aiming at her, trying to drive her away. The nurses called the psychiatrist and, with two nurses holding me down, he looked into my eyes, tried to talk to me, but I was completely deranged and psychotic. He gave me an injection, and I was carted away down the corridor to 'time out'.

On that occasion my 'time out' seemed to last for ever, hour after long hour. I saw the psychiatrist three times when he came to check me, only to give me more injections every time. Drink and food were brought in to me. And all the while I stayed huddled up on the floor in the corner, screaming because I could hear my mother and the 'voice' taunting me, even voicing my thoughts as they occurred to me.

After a very long time with no stimulation, no noise, white walls, white floor and white door to stare at, I began to calm down and went to the other extreme of deep depression. I just sobbed and sobbed, until my reservoir of tears dried up. Then I just sat on the cold tiles staring vacantly into space.

Eventually the psychiatrist came back and looked into my eyes with a penlight. He talked to me, but I could not understand what he was saying. I tried to tell him my mother hated me, that she had killed Skip, that there was nowhere safe for me. But it all burbled out an incoherent mess that didn't make any sense. He just nodded, and after a few more words, left again.

A little while after this two nurses came in, picked me up off the floor, and took me back to my room. I noticed that they had taken my cupboard and chair away, my bed now the sole item of furniture. They sat me on my bed until a male nurse took me to the bathroom and gave me a bath. Dressed in a fresh white gown, I was taken back to my room, and the door locked behind me. And through all of this, despite their efforts at conversation, I remained silent. It was as if I were in a deep trance. I sat on my bed for a long while after I had been put back in my room. Then I got up and, with uncertain steps, I went across to the window. I began to sob to myself, big tears running down my face. I didn't know it then, but I had just spent three days in 'time out'.

I stayed in my room from now on, and all my meals were brought to me. I saw the psychiatrist occasionally, but I really feared him by now. It was his say-so that determined whether I'd be put back into 'time out'.

Finally, after what seemed like an eternity, two nurses came into my room with a wheelchair. Slippers were put on my feet, and they sat me in the chair. A blanket was put over my lap; then I was wheeled out into the corridor, past the 'time-out' rooms, out through the locked ward door, into another long corridor.

One of the nurses knocked upon a door and I was wheeled into a room where two men were seated either side of a desk. To my surprise I found myself brought before my father and the psychiatrist.

'Hello, Alex,' said my father.

I just stared and stared. Was my mind playing tricks on me again? Had he come to take me home? And if I went home would my mother be there to hurt me?

I burst into tears.

'Dad,' I sobbed. 'I'm sorry, please take me home … please take me home …'

My father, with a pained expression on his face to see his son so distressed, turned his attention back to the psychiatrist.

Deep down I still had the ability to listen, even if my interaction skills were severely impaired.

'He's very seriously ill,' the psychiatrist was saying. 'His psychosis has gained complete control of him. He's totally detached from reality. I think it's the best option we've got. The drug treatment has proven ineffective. He's on as much Chlorpromazine as we dare give him, and it's not working. This is the best option left to us to break his cycle of decline …'

There were more words spoken between my father and the psychiatrist, but I missed them as my mind wandered, and I gazed around the room. Then my attention snapped back.

'He's been like this for nearly six weeks now, you know, and he's not getting any better.' said the psychiatrist. 'In fact I would say he's declining.'

Nearly six weeks he said. That really got my attention, broke through my mental barriers. I thought I'd only been here about a fortnight.

'And you are sure?' my father persisted. 'Absolutely sure ...'

'Yes,' the psychiatrist replied. 'He's suffering a severe psychotic illness. I believe it's a depressive psychosis. He's completely obsessed with the death of his dog, and he has psychotic delusions that his mother wants him dead. We have to break this cycle of decline.'

'I'm not happy about this,' my father responded.

'It's the most effective treatment we have for severe depressive illness, and it has value in the treatment of depressive psychosis. It has a high success rate.'

'What if I refuse to give my permission?'

'With respect, Mr Sinclair,' the psychiatrist replied, 'Alex is in *our* custody as a sectioned patient. I don't need your permission to conduct the electro-convulsive therapy, but I would like your support, nevertheless.'

'But ECT is so drastic,' my father persisted. 'Is there nothing else?'

'Yes, there are other drugs, Haloperidol for example. In my opinion a course of ECT to break his depressive psychosis, accompanied by treatment with Haloperidol, will result in a dramatic improvement ...'

'Dad,' I cried out, interrupting him and the psychiatrist, 'I don't want to stay here.' I decided to spill the beans to the one person in the world I trusted. 'They're horrible to me here, and I don't like it on my own all the time ...' I stifled a sob. 'Please, please, take me home ... I'll be good, I promise...'

My father turned his attention back to me. The psychiatrist looked exasperated at the interruption, but I ignored him. I reached out to my father with both my hands; my arms, thin and cold, were sticking out of the white gown that was two sizes too big for me.

I became frantic, screaming to be taken home, and the psychiatrist told the nurses to take me back to the ward.

'Daddy … Daddy … Daddy …' I screamed over and over again as I was taken away. By now I was completely hysterical as the nurses hurried me back to the ward.

As my father finished his meeting with the psychiatrist, as he drove home afterwards, I had been put back in 'time out' until I calmed down, and that was where I stayed the rest of the day. Eventually I was taken back to my room and given my tea, supervised by Nurse Harris, who stood watching as I ate my meal. Then I received my tablets, the pink syrup, and was put to bed.

When my light was turned off and I knew I was alone, I got out of bed and stood at my window staring out at the darkness. I watched as a car's headlights came on and it drove away. By now I was very drowsy, so I clambered back into bed and sobbed myself to sleep. I just wanted to go home with my father, but now that didn't seem as if it was going to happen. I'd have to undergo ECT first, whatever that entailed, before the psychiatrist would let me go…

Within a day or two of my seeing my father, I found myself put in my dressing gown and slippers, and taken downstairs to a part of the children's building I had never been to before.

As we left the ward I thought that perhaps I would see my father again, and was still wondering why he had not spent some time with me, since he had come all the way to Monmouthshire to see the psychiatrist.

The two nurses led me down a corridor to a room at the back of the building. To my unease I found myself confronted by the psychiatrist and two male nurses, who stood waiting next to a trolley-bed that had two long straps that dangled from it. Behind the trolley-bed was a contraption on a stand that looked like a big radio, with dials and switches.

I was really anxious by now as the door was closed behind me, and the nurses took my dressing gown and slippers off me. I was told to get up on the trolley and lie down. At first I resisted, but the psychiatrist put a rare smile on his face and told me not to worry. He held my hand as he helped me up on to the trolley, and said that I was to have an injection that would make me sleep for ten minutes, after which I could go back to the ward.

I nervously lay down on the trolley, and panicked at first as the two straps were done up over my chest and knees.

'There's nothing to worry about,' said the psychiatrist calmly. 'They're just to stop you falling off the trolley.'

I allowed myself to be strapped down, and anxiously watched the four nurses as they moved to the four corners of the bed. By now I was very frightened. The psychiatrist took no notice, squeezing some gel out of a tube and rubbing the cold fluid on my temples. Then, before I realised what he was doing, he'd placed a strap around my head that wired me to the 'radio'. I began to cry as he rubbed my arm with a swab, then gave me an injection and I fell asleep …

I awoke on the trolley feeling very disorientated. My arms, back, and legs ached as if I'd run ten miles. The psychiatrist smiled at me and helped me to sit up and get off the trolley; the nurses helped me on with my dressing gown and slippers. Then, with nothing said to me, I was taken from the treatment room and back upstairs to the ward.

Put back in my room, I sat on my bed as the nurses left, closing my door behind them. I felt really strange, my disorientation acute, and I was confused about where I was, my mind mixing the hospitals I'd been to over the years as a child.

A nurse came in with a glass of milk and she began to chat easily with me as if I knew her. I interrupted her, asking her name.

She smiled, replying: 'You know me, Alex. I'm Nurse Harris. Surely you've not forgotten that!'

I stared blankly at her. I *had* forgotten her name.

By the following morning my mind had recovered some of its equilibrium after a night's sleep. I was not to know it at the time, but ECT can affect the brain in adverse ways, from cognitive ability to impairing memory, and can cause cortical atrophy and fibrosis (lesions in the brain's matter, often causing physical damage that can last a lifetime). Nurse Johnson came to my room, and gave me my medication. Then she helped me on with my dressing gown and slippers, and took me to the day room. The boys were seated at the dining tables, doing written work set for them by a teacher called Mrs Howell, who came every weekday morning.

I found myself guided to an easy chair and was told to sit down. Nurse Johnson placed a few comics on the seat next to me, but I wasn't interested in the books because I still felt so disorientated. I just sat and stared into space, hands in my lap and content to stay there for the rest of the morning.

For the first time since my arrival at Pen-y-Fal I was allowed to have lunch with the other boys seated at the tables. Directly after lunch, I was given my tablets and returned to my room, where I lay on my bed and dozed for the rest of the afternoon.

From now on, every second day, two nurses took me down to the treatment room where the psychiatrist waited with his trolley and 'radio'. Of course, I didn't know what was being done to me at the time. Had I been able to see my treatment for myself, I would have beheld four nurses holding down a flailing child having to all appearances an epileptic-type seizure.

By the time a fortnight had passed and I had received half my treatment (six ECTs), my belief that my mother wanted me dead began to diminish, driven by force out of my brain, along with the 'voice' that had taunted me. However, I became very confused, and daily found myself asking the nurses the same questions – Who were they? What day was it? Where was I? They would smile at me and remind me of their names, and answer my questions. Slowly, but inexorably, as my treatment proceeded my brain was being adversely affected, regardless of the benefits of the 'cure'.

While I was being treated by ECT in March I did not see my father at all, despite daily pleas to the nurses to telephone him. The nurses always nodded and said they'd ring him, but he never came, and I convinced myself that he had abandoned me. The thought of being abandoned is a terrible thing to any child, but particularly one who is mentally fragile. As it had happened to me in Greece, it had the potential to cause me real fear and panic. In the end I came to believe that he did not want to come, and became very despondent. I was not to know it, but my father was far away during March 1976, busy again in the Middle East acting as an emissary for the Israeli Prime Minister to the Egyptians.

With the arrival of April I had made remarkable progress in my recovery. The treatment by ECT had ended by now and my psychosis was largely eliminated. How much of my recovery was due to my medication change from Chlorpromazine to Haloperidol can only be guessed. All I knew was that at some point near the end of March I was no longer taunted by the 'voice', and my mother all but ceased to shout commands at me.

With this newfound mental equilibrium, my existence at Pen-y-Fal improved. I now spent all day in the day room, and was encouraged to sit at the table during the mornings to participate in simple lessons given by Mrs Howell.

I had regular meetings with the psychiatrist, and he'd ask me how I was. Was I still afraid of my mother? Had she been shouting commands at me again? Had the 'voice' been talking to me?

With my mental state nearly restored, I now realised it was in my interest to deny everything. An admission that I'd heard my mother or the 'voice' would set me back. It was better to deny everything, regardless of whether I *was* still occasionally hearing my mother, *was* still frightened of her, because then the psychiatrist would keep me at Pen-y-Fal longer.

By the beginning of April I'd managed to convince the psychiatrist that I was much better. This meant I was finally allowed to move from my single room into one of the six-bed dormitories. This was a great improvement, for I had begun to make a few friends on the ward.

One afternoon I was sitting on my bed reading a book when the door opened and Nurse Harris showed in a boy of about twelve. He was very distressed and evidently mentally ill because he kept flinching and glancing behind him.

I know, I thought, you're hearing voices. I had become adept at recognising the symptoms of my own illness in others.

Nurse Harris placed the boy's holdall on the vacant bed opposite mine.

'Alex,' Nurse Harris said. 'This is Brian. He's not very well at the moment and is a bit upset because he's not been here before. You'll look after him, won't you?'

I gave my assent, before turning my attention back to my book, knees tucked under my chin.

Nurse Harris told Brian that tea would not be long, that it was served at five o'clock in the day room, and then she left.

Brian sat sniffling on his bed, as distraught as I had originally been to end up here. Determined to remain aloof, I ignored him.

I had been reading for just a few minutes when the door opened and a boy named Mark came in. Mark was a blond fifteen-year-old I'd not had much to do with because he was older than me, and I knew he was a bit aggressive. I'd never talked to him, yet he'd been at Pen-y-Fal ever since I'd arrived.

Mark stared at Brian, then leapt across the room and threw Brian off his bed on to the floor, screaming and shouting that Brian had taken his friend's bed. His friend had been John, a boy who had gone home a few days before.

Frightened and not about to get involved in a scrap with a boy a lot bigger than me, I quickly backed up into the corner of my bed against the wall, just as Nurse Harris rushed into the room to see what the commotion was. Mark was very agitated by now, shouting at the terrified Brian, who lay crying on the floor. Nurse Harris called for help, and Mr Thomas, the male nurse, came running into the room. They put out placating hands, trying to calm Mark down.

'Come on, Mark,' Mr Thomas said firmly. 'You know John went home a few days ago. This is Brian's bed now.'

Mark paused, arms in the air, silent and suddenly pacified. A blank look came over his face. He put his arms down, and allowed Mr Thomas to take his hand and lead him from the room.

Nurse Harris picked a shaking Brian up off the floor, sat him down on his bed, and sat next to him, talking and calming him down. Brian had been terrified by the attack.

It reaffirmed to me the fact that psychiatric units, even those for children, were not without the risk of attack from an unstable patient, unless staff were present all the time to intervene. Even though I had been very ill, I had never been aggressive to others and was more likely to hurt myself; that didn't necessarily go for the other boys.

A few days later I was sitting in the day room watching a western on the television, my fear of TVs having subsided in proportion to my recovery, when Mark came and sat next to me.

'Hello,' he said. 'What's the film?'

'Only some western,' I answered, hoping he was not going to be aggressive towards me.

'Oh yes,' he responded amiably. 'What's the action?'

'Well, there are these gunslingers in town, and the sheriff's just about to shoot them ...'

Mark nodded, and continued to talk as we watched the film. To my amazement, far from being a big thug, he turned out to be well educated, and very chatty. He talked all afternoon, telling me about his father, who owned a car dealership in Monmouth, and his mother, who was in something called the Inner Wheel.

'She hasn't got any time for me though,' he grumbled. 'She's always too busy with her friends. Then they sent me to this place, and I can't go home ...'

I suppose I fell into the trap. I responded, telling him

about my life and my parents, that my mother hated me. The conversation flowed all afternoon, and I was astonished to learn Mark had been at Pen-y-Fal nearly *two* years. Eventually, I broached the subject that was lurking at the back of my mind. I asked him why he was at Pen-y-Fal.

'The doctor says I've got a severe personality disorder – schizophrenia. Why are you here?'

'A psychotic illness …'

'I hate the doctor,' Mark said after a moment's silence.

'Me too.'

Mark flashed me a winning smile, as if I'd just passed a test.

I found that I had made an unlikely friend. It just goes to prove that you can't judge a book by its cover, I thought.

A few days later Nurse Harris stopped me in the corridor. She'd noticed me spending a lot of time with Mark, and wanted a quiet word. She asked me if I was happy to be friends with Mark. He hadn't threatened me, had he? she asked. I shook my head. Nurse Harris nodded.

'Okay,' she said, 'but be careful. Don't tell him much about yourself,' she warned me.

Wide-eyed, I asked why.

'Mark is very unstable,' she told me. She stole a glance over her shoulder as if she should not be telling me this. 'He's a sociopath,' she confided; 'that means he uses people and he is very unpredictable.' She reminded me about what happened to Brian.

With that final caution, Nurse Harris sent me back to the day room. Mark beckoned me across to the television. There was a film on, and he had kept a seat for me. I sat down as he, grinning, turned his attention back to the television. I sat mulling over what Nurse Harris had told me. Her warning not to tell Mark about myself resonated with my conversation with him that first afternoon. I had already done precisely what Nurse Harris warned me not to do. I stared discreetly out of the side of my eye at Mark.

Surely he couldn't be as dangerous as that? Could he?

There was a small pretty nurse on Ward 3 called Nurse Clark. When I had been psychotic and placed in 'time out' it had often been her duty to keep an eye on me. She had seen me at my worst – screaming my head off and huddled on the floor in the corner. Now I was sort of proud of myself that I was getting better, and tried to be polite to all the nurses at every opportunity, determined to send the message via the nurses to the psychiatrist that I was better and could go home soon.

One morning I was sitting at the table with Mrs Howell, who was giving us a maths lesson, when Nurse Clark came over and told me to follow her. Glad for any break from lessons, I followed her from the day room. We went down the corridor, and she took me through the locked ward door into the main building, and then downstairs. I had always come this way for my ECT. However, instead of the usual corridors, the nurse took me to the front of the building, and showed me into a room with a few chairs and tables.

To my immense joy, there stood my father, looking out of the window. I flew across the room and flung my arms around him. What immediately struck me was that my father was very deeply tanned and healthy-looking.

For the next hour I chatted to my father, and he seemed really pleased that I had made a substantial recovery. He apologised that he had not been to visit me, explaining that the psychiatrist had asked him not to come while I was being treated, and then his work had taken him to the Middle East for three weeks.

All too soon a nurse appeared, telling me that it was time for me to return to the ward for lunch. In parting, I pleaded with my father to ask the psychiatrist if I could go home soon. My father nodded, and as I left with the nurse he told me that he had an appointment to see the psychiatrist after our meeting.

I went back to the ward with a bounce in my step, convinced that I would be going home within just a few days.

On my return to the ward, everyone was already sat at the tables for lunch. Mark waved to me that he had kept a seat next to his for lunch.

'Well?' he asked as soon as I sat down. 'What's up?'

I told him excitedly that my father had visited me, and that he'd said he was going to meet the psychiatrist to see if I could go home. If I had expected a normal response, I was suddenly made aware that Mark was very unstable.

'You're leaving me here!' he screamed in insane fury. 'You're going to leave me like everyone else always does.'

My mind suddenly flashed to the warning words of Nurse Harris.

Mark leapt up from his seat, picked up his meal of cottage

pie, and in rage hurled the plate across the room. He began to scream and shout, throwing his chair around.

The male nurse rushed across and together with Nurse Harris grabbed Mark. His destination, I guessed, would be 'time out' for the rest of the afternoon.

It was at this point I suddenly felt very strange, dizzy, and disorientated in a way I'd never felt before ...

The next thing I remember is waking up on the floor. Nurse Johnson was holding me as I lay on my side, and she was talking softly to me, telling me everything was going to be all right. My mind was very muddled. I was picked up off the floor and sat in an easy chair. Nurse Johnson held my hand, and kept telling me I was going to be fine. She asked me if I had ever had fits before. Was I epileptic? Dazed, I shook my head and asked what had happened.

Nurse Johnson knelt before me, and told me not to be frightened, but I had had an epileptic fit, a loss of consciousness with a spasmodic seizure.

I could feel my hair prickling on the back of my neck. Epilepsy. The word had terrifying connotations for me. Nikki had been epileptic. He had died in my arms, and I'd never got over his traumatic loss. I broke down into quiet tears, remembering my friend.

Nurse Johnson took me to my room and told me to lie on my bed and sleep for a few hours. I was okay, she reassured me. I had just been very upset by Mark. Nevertheless, she said, she would ask the psychiatrist to come and see me to check me over. I lay down, thoughts of poor Nikki running through my head, and eventually dozed off.

The psychiatrist came to visit me that afternoon. He tested my reflexes and looked into my eyes. He was concerned that I had suffered an epileptic fit, and instructed Nurse Johnson to keep an eye on me for the next few days.

The meeting with my father and my petit mal occurred on a Friday afternoon and I had not seen Mark again that day. They kept him in 'time out' for the rest of the afternoon, and as a consequence of his aggressive behaviour moved him that same day from his six-bed dorm to a room on his own, so they could lock his door at night.

For the rest of that weekend I steered away from Mark, and he shot me angry looks. I was sorry because he'd become my friend.

On Monday I was due to see the psychiatrist, and I knew he'd take the decision whether I could go home, or have to stay another few weeks at Pen-y-Fal. I was desperate to go home by now, despite a deep-seated fear of my mother. I had been at Pen-y-Fal since the beginning of January, a total of fifteen weeks.

My Monday-morning meeting with the psychiatrist came and, very nervously, I sat in his office while he talked to me. He asked me how I felt. Had I heard the 'voice' or my mother again? No, I declared, I no longer heard anything.

Did I still believe my mother hated me and wanted me dead? The psychiatrist asked.

This was a difficult one for me, for my mother had proved by her actions that this fact was true.

Again I shook me head, telling the psychiatrist I was sorry for being so confused when I was ill.

After a range of similar questions, the psychiatrist sat back in his chair, and I awaited the verdict. In the end he gave me a rare smile. Okay, he said finally. He was concerned that I'd had an epileptic seizure, so he wanted me to stay on the ward a few days more, but I could go home on Friday.

I was utterly overwhelmed at this news and, filled with excitement, went with the nurse back to the ward, where I sought Brian out and told him I was going home at the end of the week. Aware of how Mark had reacted when I'd told him I was going home soon, I avoided him as he sat scowling at the television.

Envy is a terrible thing, especially in a person as unstable as Mark, and I thought, 'All I have to do is avoid him for the rest of the week. Five days more, and I'll be safely on my way home with my father.' But then I'd have my mother to contend with, and the realisation of this fact took the edge off my joy that afternoon.

I spent the rest of the week at Pen-y-Fal counting off the hours and days. Now, during lessons and meals, I contrived to sit at the other table from Mark, who no longer kept a seat for me. Instead, I noticed him scowling as I talked to Brian, who, being in my dormitory and my age, I had become friends with; in Brian I had found a kindred spirit in a boy who suffered a similar illness to mine.

After an eternally long Thursday afternoon and evening, Friday morning came and I threw my clothes into my holdall, all squashed in pell-mell as I struggled to do up the zip. Brian sat on his bed talking while I concluded my business of getting ready to go home, then the two of us went to the day room.

We had only been in the day room for twenty minutes, frustratingly made to sit at the tables for morning lessons, when Nurse Harris came and told me that my father had telephoned the ward office to say he would collect me at two o'clock. In exasperation I returned to my maths lesson.

Why couldn't he come sooner? I wondered.

'Never mind,' said Brian, seated next to me. 'You'll be going home today. By this evening you'll be at home, and back in your own room.'

I flashed him a smile. He was right, of course. What did four hours matter after nearly four months in this place?

No one will ever know precisely what took place next, for it happened with such rapidity that it took everyone by surprise. My attention was on my work when out of the corner of my eye I caught a flash of movement. Mark had got up from his seat as if to go to the toilet, but instead pounced on Brian.

With an insane shout of 'You've stolen my friend!' he threw Brian on to the floor and before anyone could intervene, stabbed Brian in the eye with a sharpened pencil.

Brian let out a tortured scream, and two nurses pounced on Mark to drag him off the injured twelve-year-old.

My overwhelming memory is of blood all over Brian's face and oozing between his fingers as he lay on the floor holding his eye. Mr Thomas rushed across to help drag Mark away as he shouted and flailed wildly. Nurses Johnson and Harris hurriedly produced a folded towel, which they held on Brian's face as he sobbed in agony, and was taken away to where he could receive medical attention.

Mrs Howell abandoned the lessons that day. Everyone was too traumatised by what had happened, and I was shaken too. What if Mark had attacked me? I would now be in Brian's predicament. There had been so much blood and screaming and he'd lost an eye.

Everyone was kept in the day room for the rest of the day. Mark was not far away, for I could hear him shouting abuse at the staff as they kept him securely locked up in 'time out'. I had never realised how dangerous Mark really was. I kept looking at the wall clock, counting off the hours and minutes until my father came to take me away from this suddenly dangerous place. We boys ate a subdued lunch, Brian's empty chair next to mine emphasising the horror of what had happened.

Eventually, at 2.30 p.m., Nurse Clark came to the day room and called me. My father had arrived, she said, and was waiting for me downstairs. I hurried to my dorm to collect my holdall, and set off down the corridor with the nurse.

While Nurse Clark's attention was taken as she fumbled in her pocket for the keys to the ward door, I darted across to the 'time out' door, and peered in through the small window. Mark was standing, clad in a white gown and bare-foot in the middle of the room. He had been sedated. We stared at each other for a long moment. Then I made a final bid for peace, some form of reconciliation: I placed my hand on the glass. After a long moment, he came over to the door and placed his hand on the glass to mirror mine. We stared at each other.

'Alex! Come away from there!' Nurse Clark ordered.

I blinked away tears of sorrow for Mark. They'd never let him go home now. I gave him a smile that he didn't return, then turned and walked away, out of Ward 3, and downstairs to my father.

CHAPTER 13

In Mortal Peril

The June sunshine streamed in through the French doors at my grandmother's house as we sat for Sunday lunch. It was my thirteenth birthday and I'd had a wonderful day so far, pleased with my presents, and happy in anticipation, for my parents had invited two of my friends from Kings – Peanut and a boy called David – to my house for a birthday tea.

My father was more content than I had seen him for a long time, at ease that my mother was going through a more reasonable phase, but I knew that her moods were as changeable as the weather. Today she was nice; but tomorrow?

I had returned home in April 1976 to a much more settled house than I'd left in January. My mother had even smiled as I came in the front door, but I noticed her smile didn't reach her eyes; they remained cold mica behind her spectacles, bereft of humanity. Despite this she was kind to me on my arrival at home, something that had taken me by complete surprise. The spring of 1976 was one of my mother's rare periods of moderation, when she tried to be pleasant – so long as things were going her way. She was very pleased that in addition to his salary from the university, my father was making a lot of money out of the Israelis, money my parents jokingly called Dad's 'retirement fund'.

There was, however, a fly in the ointment. I hardly recognised the house, although I retained some dreamlike memories of it. Also, confronted with the reality that Ingrid was a lively three-year-old, I became very upset because I hardly recognised her; my memory of her was that she was little more than a baby. Outwardly restored to sanity and no longer psychotic, it now became apparent that my mind had been affected by the illness, my memory damaged by the ECT.

During my treatment I had always returned to the ward very disorientated, and sometimes not recognised the nurses or my friends. By the time twenty-four hours had passed my memory had always begun to recover. However, it was only another twenty-four hours before the psychiatrist had given me another dose of ECT, and then the whole frightening process had started again.

My parents could do nothing that first weekend of my return home, except be very patient, calmly show me the house, hope to jog my memory; they almost had to reintroduce Ingrid to me.

On Monday morning my father was on the telephone to the psychiatrist to express his consternation that my memory had been damaged. The psychiatrist told my father not to be overly concerned. It was a common side effect, he said, but he had not realised it extended to my more deep-seated memories. It would just take time and patience to refamiliarise me with my memories, memories that had been 'whited' from my mind, as he clinically termed it. My father was far from satisfied; indeed, he was very concerned. My mother listened to all my father told her, then told him that at least I was no longer psychotic. If this was the cost of cure, she said, then it was just something they would have to persevere with.

In the days ahead my mother had found opportunities to ask me about the past. Did I remember living in Falmouth? Did I remember the time I had fallen and broken my arm? She always asked me these questions when my father was not present. Subtly, slowly, she began to ask me questions about our latter years in Cornwall. I realised she was building up to something, and within a few days she revealed her hand. She asked me if I remembered living with her in Athens.

Although my memory was very muddled – certain of my memories 'whited' – I *did* remember living with her in Athens. She had abused me dreadfully. Indeed, I was still having nightmares about my experiences at her hands in Greece, about my time in the asylum. However, despite all that had happened to me, I was aware that I shouldn't let on just how much I remembered. I realised it was safer to deny remembering most of these events, so I pretended my memory was more damaged than it really was. If my mother ever realised I remembered she had abused and nearly killed me in Greece, then I knew she had the potential to be very dangerous indeed.

There was a second problem that made itself manifest within a few days of my return home, and that was my petits mals – the minor epileptic episodes when I lost consciousness for a few minutes – sometimes with mild spasmodic seizures.

It must have seemed to my parents that I had been returned with more problems than I had been admitted with, albeit of a different nature.

I was immediately taken to be examined by our GP, and after some brief auto-responsive tests, he said he was sure there was no brain abnormality or illness; it was most likely the result of the ECT. He told my father that so long as my seizures remained only slight, there was nothing to be alarmed about.

Once again my father telephoned the psychiatrist at Pen-y-Fal, who confirmed that I had suffered a seizure on the ward, and reluctantly conceded it may have been triggered by the ECT. There were pros and cons to the treatment, he said, and petits mals were a very uncommon side effect; they would probably cease as suddenly as they had started. My father came off the telephone outraged at the psychiatrist's attitude, and declared that he would never let him near me ever again.

Because it was clear to my parents that I was not completely recovered, and still in a frail mental state, I was not sent to school for the summer term. My father was adamant he wanted something better for me than education at a special school, and even my mother agreed that my attendance at Meadowbank was a complete waste of time. Now that my father was earning a very good supplementary income from the Israelis for his work as a foreign affairs adviser, he decided to send me back to Kings in the autumn. It was a decision supported by Sally Martin. She now interceded by accompanying my father to visit the headmaster of Kings to press the point that it had been concluded while I was at Pen-y-Fal that I was not autistic at all, and never had been. It would therefore be better for me to attend a private school that could make provision for my delicate mental state. After a long meeting, the headmaster agreed to admit me to Kings in September.

In August 1976, my father left again for the Middle East, his destination a briefing in Jerusalem, to be followed by a series of meetings in Israel and Egypt.

While my father was away my life with Mother wavered between uncertainty and the constant possibility of unpleasantness or even violence. My father had only been gone two days when my mother telephoned Sally Martin to ask if I could be placed in respite for a fortnight. However, my mother's machinations were completely undone this time. Sally Martin responded that I had that spring spent four months in hospital, where I'd been assessed as not autistic. I was therefore ineligible to be sent to Ely Hospital, and so there was no placement that was suitable; my best interests would thus be served by peace and quiet at home.

During the ferocious heat wave that summer of 1976, which daily reached temperatures of 32°C, I was forbidden to go out, often treated with contempt by my mother, and threatened with a good hiding if I didn't obey her. And so I existed in this atmosphere for a fortnight, terrified of her, for I knew she was capable of great evil. One day I was merely walking down the hall when she flew out of the kitchen, screaming obscenities at me, and began slapping my face, before throwing me against the wall. With the salty taste of blood in my mouth from a split lip, my only defence was non-response, just to go limp on the floor. I knew that to fight back would only provoke greater violence. The next thing I remember is waking up on the floor, feeling disorientated and sick; apparently I'd had another epileptic fit.

As a result of this incident my mother took me to see our GP. All I could do was stand by and listen while she told the doctor that I was suffering epileptic fits. She lied, telling the doctor that I'd been collapsing with severe seizures once every day or two, and that on the last occasion I'd bruised my face and split my lip. The doctor was very concerned as he listened to all this, and after a careful examination – looking into my eyes, testing my reflexes – told my mother that he was still sure there was no brain abnormality. He would nevertheless put me on an anti-epileptic drug called Phenobarbitone. This is a powerful barbiturate, the doctor warned; it should therefore be used with care and moderation. A small dose once a day would limit the seizures; they should be less frequent, less severe, and swifter in passing.

My mother came away from the consultation with a curious expression of satisfaction on her face. I was sure she was once again moving towards some as yet unknown objective. That very same day, as soon as we got home, she gave me several tablets. I knew I was supposed to only take one, but they were forced upon me, and I spent the rest of the day very sleepy. The Phenobarbitone was given to me in large quantities for the next few days, my waking world one of sedation in which I was too pacified to do anything at all.

Then, as suddenly as it had started, my mother's application of this medication to me ceased. Her experimentation had ended. It didn't take me long to realise why my mother had suddenly stopped forcing the pills on me. My father returned from the Middle East, and my mother did not want him to know what she had been doing.

My mother quite openly told my father that she had taken me to the doctor, and that he had placed me on Phenobarbitone, telling him that I had been suffering major fits. I don't think it was true. Yes, I had occasionally suffered petits mals, and fainted. However, in the month that followed my father only saw me suffer two minor attacks. What no one realised by that autumn was that my mother was stock-piling Phenobarbitone, a repeat prescription, dose by dose, until she was in possession of a very substantial – and dangerous – quantity indeed.

At the beginning of September I went back to Kings, this time into 3B. On the basis that the psychiatrist had assessed that I was not autistic, my father and Sally Martin persuaded the headmaster that I should be moved up a grade. I was still far behind the other boys because I had missed so much education in recent years due to my illness. However, I went into 3B, and to my pleasure found myself in the same class as Peanut, with whom I now spent every day.

Within just a fortnight of my return to Kings, my father secretly arranged with Margaret Nutt that he would pick up Peanut on the way to school in the mornings, as Kings was located not far from the university. Now, at the age of thirteen, Peanut and I returned home in the afternoons on the bus. My mother, ignorant of my father's arrangement with Margaret, was quite happy for my father to take me to school in the mornings and for me to catch a bus home at the end of the day. She was engrossed looking after Ingrid, who had now started kindergarten, and taking and collecting Vicky from school.

My mother's calm mood persisted through the early autumn of that year. There is no doubt, however, that she would have gone into an insane rage if she had discovered that my father had resumed the school-run with Margaret Nutt.

My grandmother, Margaret Nutt and Peanut, and my parents, all lived within half a mile of each other in the quiet suburb of Fairwater, separated by just a few streets. It was an autumn in which I was allowed more freedom than I had ever known before, permitted to wander at will on the weekends to visit my grandmother and Peanut. However, my mother's period of calm was not to last.

Towards the end of October there came one Sunday morning when my parents let me walk to my grandmother's house to mow her lawn. As it happened, when I arrived I found Uncle Tom there, and he'd already mowed the grass.

As I was not needed by my grandmother that morning, I decided to go to visit Peanut, where I spent the morning.

Then Margaret asked if I'd like to stay for lunch, to which I said I would like to, knowing my parents did not expect me back before four o'clock, assuming I'd have lunch with my grandmother. I stayed to lunch, spent the afternoon with Peanut, and arrived back home a little after four.

On my arrival at home, I found that my parents had had a terrible row over some slight imagined by my mother. It did not take much to send her into a fierce rage. As soon as I walked in the door, I knew that there was trouble, for my mother flew at me, grabbing me painfully, and shaking me, asking where I had been. She had rung my grandmother at lunchtime, only to find I was not there. Terrified of her, I admitted I had spent the day with Peanut. Mere mention of the Nutts was like a red rag to a bull to my mother. She turned on my father, asking if he had known I was going to Margaret Nutt's house. Of course, my dad, innocent as he was, denied any knowledge.

My mother, in an insane rage by now, began screaming, throwing dishes about the kitchen, and accusing my father of sleeping with Margaret Nutt. Of course, there was no truth in this, but the very fact that my father had secretly reinstated the school-run placed him on the defensive. He lost his temper and stormed out of the house, got in his car, and drove away, believing it best to extricate himself from the situation until my mother calmed down.

Once my father was gone my mother turned on me, demanding to know if my father was secretly seeing Margaret Nutt. I denied everything, but my mother was not so easily put off. She began pushing me around the kitchen, and this culminated in her throwing me bodily against the wall with a resounding bang. Once I would have dissolved into tears, but now at the age of thirteen I just picked myself up off the floor, refusing to rise to her bait. However, in getting up I had challenged my mother, something she could not tolerate. As I rose, I suddenly felt the cold steel of a carving knife held across my throat. I gulped in terror at the expression on her face. Again, she asked me if my father had known I was going to Peanut's house, and again I denied it. My mother blinked slowly, almost reptile-like, then before I could react, she kneed me viciously in the groin. I screamed in agony, and collapsed to the floor in tears. My mother seemed satisfied with that response and, showing as much emotion as if she'd been swatting a fly, let go of me and walked away, leaving me to crawl from the kitchen.

My mother remained in an insane rage for the next few days, refusing to cook for my father and me, and just looked after Vicky and Ingrid. She was beginning, I think, to realise the time was approaching – with my increasing age – when she would be powerless to terrify and control me, and my father was also becoming resolved not to give in to her any more. On this occasion my father just brazened it out, making our own breakfasts, and taking me out for fish and chips every evening for the next week, until my mother gave in and began to cook for the whole family once again.

October ended with a return to an uneasy sort of normality, only now the family had split into two 'armed' camps – my mother and Vicky on the one hand, and my father and I on the other. In an effort to defuse the situation my father decided to cease the school-run with Margaret until the onset of winter. I now only saw Peanut in school.

At the beginning of November my father took me to see my psychiatrist, Dr Evans at Whichurch Hospital. Dr Evans declared himself satisfied with my progress. He was pleased that I had returned to school, pleased too that my mental equilibrium had returned. There was no sign of any psychotic disorder, although I would have to keep taking Haloperidol for the next few years to ensure there was no recurrence of the illness. He was more concerned that I was still suffering debilitating flashbacks and nightmares about my time in Greece, remarking that I might suffer this post-traumatic stress disorder for many years to come. There was one matter that Dr Evans was very insistent about, and that was that I must never be subjected to such trauma ever again. If this were to occur it might well trigger another psychotic illness, only next time, he warned my father, it had the potential to be much more damaging.

In mid-November, my father was notified by the Israelis that they wanted him to conduct diplomatic talks in Cairo. This work was to take him away for two weeks, he told my mother, and he announced that he would be departing within a few days.

'I don't care what you do,' my mother spat. 'Go if you want to.'

My father tried to be reasonable, pointing out that the

money he was being paid would be very welcome, would add significantly to their 'retirement fund'.

My mother considered this for a long moment, and one could almost see the calculation taking place behind her cold obsidian eyes, as she weighed in the balance the fact that she was fanatical in her desire for money, whatever its source. In the end she nodded her assent, and I could almost see the relief in my father, the way his shoulders relaxed.

Within just a few days my father, case packed and brief-case in car, was gone, and I again found myself alone with my mother and sisters. However, my fear of my mother had again subsided, and despite her violent behaviour in October I believed she had returned to a state of normality. I was wrong.

My father had only been gone a few days when Peanut suggested that instead of going to school on my own by bus while my dad was away, as my parents wanted, it was a better idea for me to walk to his house every morning. His mother would then take us both to school and collect us at the end of the school day. It didn't take me long to accept his offer as it was no fun waiting at bus stops in the rain on cold November mornings and afternoons. After all, I thought, if I was careful my mother would never find out.

For the next week I quite happily left the house at the normal time, but instead of waiting for the bus in the street, I walked to Peanut's house and was taken to school with him in Margaret's Mini. This all proceeded well for the first few days, and I was satisfied by the thought that I was saving my bus fare, money I used at lunchtime in the local sweet shop.

Monday, 22 November, was a wet and windy day, so I was very pleased when Peanut and I came out of school at the end of the day to find Margaret waiting in her car to take us home. The journey home was unremarkable, and Peanut and I were chatting in the back of the car when we stopped at traffic lights on the outskirts of Fairwater. As we were talking I happened to glance out of the window at the car next to us, and found myself staring in stunned shock directly into my mother's face as she sat in her car looking directly at me. Then the lights changed, and the cars moved apart.

From the expression on my mother's face I realised I was in terrible trouble. I had no choice, however, except to go home and face the music. Margaret Nutt tried to bolster me when we arrived back at her house; she offered to take me home and make the excuse that I'd lost my bus fare. I knew it was no good. Margaret's presence would only inflame the situation, probably even cause problems for my father too, when he returned from the Middle East. So I trudged home in the pouring rain, cold, wet, and very frightened about what was going to happen. If she only shouted at me, I thought, I could take that, so long as she doesn't become violent. I knew I would have to face up to deceiving her about the fact that Peanut's mother had been bringing me home from school.

As soon as I opened the front door, my mother flew at me. She screamed, she shouted, she tore my satchel from me and threw it down the hallway. There was no sign of Vicky or Ingrid. They had been banished upstairs to their bedrooms while my mother took out her anger on me.

I tried to respond that I'd done no harm; Peanut was just my friend, and as it was a wet afternoon his mother had offered to give me a lift home.

'Don't tell me those lies!' my mother screamed. 'She's seeing your father in secret, isn't she!'

I denied this vehemently; after all it was untrue. Yes, they had resumed sharing the school-run, but that was all. However, this was something I dared not reveal to my mother. She was so unstable she'd claim they were having an affair, which was not true.

'Tell me the truth,' my mother shouted. 'They're plotting against me, aren't they? Tell me! Tell me! Tell me!'

I shook my head, by now terrified of her. If I'd been a bigger thirteen-year-old, perhaps things might have happened differently, perhaps I'd have been able to defend myself. But I wasn't, and my mother was about to get violent.

She threw me against the wall, and began to lay into me. I was slapped across the face very hard a number of times. I could taste blood in my mouth from where she split my lip. She bunched a fist and walloped me squarely and very pain-fully in the eye, punched me in the temple so hard I saw stars. By now I was beginning to panic. I'd never seen her so violent before, and her face, contorted in insane rage, was terrifying to behold.

Grabbing me by my hair, she dragged me upstairs to my room and threw me in through the doorway. She was gone just a few moments before she returned with a handful of tablets, which she forced me to take. By now I was very frightened, for I knew the evil she was capable of should the notion take her.

However, instead of further violence, my mother announced I would not get any tea, and I was to stay in my room until she decided what to do with me. And with that she was gone, locking my bedroom door behind her.

I awoke at six on Tuesday morning. I had been awake most of the night, my rumbling stomach reminding me I'd not eaten anything since the previous lunchtime. At the first hint of dawn, a vivid weal of red on a cloud-covered horizon, I got dressed in my school uniform. I was already dressed when I began to hear the house stir, Ingrid calling to Mum, and our mother talking to Vicky on the landing before they descended the stairs for breakfast.

I remained in my room until eventually my door was unlocked and my mother appeared. There was a complete look of hatred on her face, her eyes cold, unyielding, and full of venom.

She had to take Vicky to school and Ingrid to kindergarten, she announced, but once she had done that she was going to confront Margaret Nutt. She would not countenance that 'bitch' interfering in our family, she declared, and she would end the 'affair' with my father once and for all. And with that she was gone, slamming my bedroom door shut and locking it behind her.

I sat staring at the door for long minutes, alarmed at the disaster I had caused by my deceit, the terrible problems my father would have to face upon his return from the Middle East. I looked at myself in the mirror. I had a stunning black eye, split lip, and bruised face and temple from my mother's frenzied attack. I looked a total wreck, and suspected my mother did not want to send me to school all beaten up because of the questions that would be asked.

Despite her ability to inflict pain and terror on me, my mother was at heart an unstable person, frightened of the authorities, wary of my father's anger if he saw me in such a state. In the past she'd usually tried to cause me pain without outward signs of violence. I was not mentally ill any more, and with my increasing age she was less able to claim I had inflicted these injuries on myself. This time she had gone too far, and I think she knew it. I wouldn't be seeing anyone until my wounds had healed.

I heard the front door slam and then silence, so I knew she'd left to take Vicky and Ingrid to school. I continued to stare at myself in the mirror, unable to drag my eyes away from the damaged individual staring back at me.

My mother was gone a long time that morning, and did not return home until well past eleven. Her return was heralded by a distant slam of the front door, and my fear instantly returned to make a pit of anxiety deep in my stomach.

Had she confronted Margaret Nutt? I wondered. If she had, what had happened?

Margaret was a kind and soft sort of person, and since I had known her I'd never seen her short-tempered or even get annoyed. My mother, by contrast, was capable of terrifying rages and violence. I could only imagine the showdown that must have taken place on Margaret Nutt's doorstep. At the time I was convinced it was all my fault.

I put my book away, and sat on my bed awaiting the next development. I did not have long to wait.

I heard my mother coming up the stairs, and within moments she was in my room.

'Come with me,' she snapped.

I followed her downstairs into the sitting room, where she turned on me with great fury on her face.

She screamed, she shouted, she threw cushions about the room. Fearing another beating, I backed into the corner. I had never really seen her like this before. It was as if she was powerless in the face of my perfidy, my friendship with Peanut and Margaret. I could tell she was utterly convinced that Margaret and my father were having an affair, plotting against her; indeed, she screamed it at me, her face just inches from mine as I stood with my back hard against the wall. I gathered she had been to confront Margaret, and got no satisfaction despite all her fury and the insane rages she was capable of.

She grabbed me, and shook me hard, screaming that it was all my fault. I was the cause of all the upset in the family; I was the real cause of her inability to keep her husband. With that she threw me to the floor and gave me a terrific kick in the side, knocking all the wind out of me; I wondered if she'd cracked or broken a rib, such was the pain.

She stormed out of the room to return within minutes clutching several bottles of tablets – primarily Phenobarbitone, but also Haloperidol – and a large glass of water. Placing them on the coffee table, she grabbed me by the scruff of the neck and dragged me across the floor, to where she pinned me against the sofa.

'I hate you! I hate you! I hate you ...' she screamed.

She grabbed a bottle and began pouring tablets into my mouth, forcing me to swallow water as she crammed more and more tablets into my mouth. I coughed and spluttered; pleaded with her to stop, but she took no notice. Once one bottle was empty, she grabbed the second, and the whole process started again. Then she grabbed the third bottle, and I struggled futilely against her until all the tablets were gone.

'I hate you,' she shouted, striking me hard across the face and throwing me down to the floor. 'You'll never get in the way again, I'll make sure of it this time ... You should have stayed put away in an asylum where your sort belong!'

I began to cry in terror of her, for I knew that my time had come. She'd given me so many tablets I knew it must be fatal. I just lay on the floor gasping for breath, for I had been forced to take so many tablets, water poured into me, that I had hardly been able to breathe. I tried to get up, tried to get away from her before it was too late, but she dealt me a hard kick in the side, again knocking all the wind out of me. I returned to my prone position, curled up on the floor and unable to do anything, except to think, 'This is the end of the road. I'm going to die and my dad's not here ...'

My mother stood over me, foot on my back to hold me down, as slowly, inexorably, after about ten to fifteen minutes my thoughts became disjointed and ever more muddled; I began to slip into unconsciousness. I stared across the floor through the French doors at the garden, thinking: 'This is it. This is the last thing you're ever going see.'

Hard hands propelled me down long corridors and I screamed in anguish, screamed in fear of what was to come. A man in a white jacket ran ahead, and the big door was opened to reveal a dingy concrete room. My eyes adjusted to the darkness and I beheld a pale form on the floor, that of a naked child laying on his back, perfectly still. Deep down I knew Nikki was dead as I knelt next to him. I took hold of his hand, icy cold and stiff. I leaned forward to look into his thin pale face, took in his delicate features, the small aquiline nose. I stared for long moments, full of sorrow, and could feel my deep anguish at his death. Suddenly his eyes opened, and he stared back at me. He opened his mouth and began to laugh – my mother's laugh, at once insane and evil. I began to scream, and it went on and on …

I could feel hands holding me, warm hands that held me, shook me awake, and I opened my eyes to see the nurse holding my hand, a compassionate expression on her young face.

'It's okay, Alex,' she said. 'You're safe now. No one's going to hurt you.'

How could I tell her it was my nightmare? I rolled on to my side, turning my face away from her, and sobbed to myself.

I had been in hospital over a week, and it was only in the

last few days that I had been aware enough to learn I was in the University Hospital of Wales, where I was being treated for the massive barbiturate overdose that had almost taken my life.

When I had been brought in I had been unconscious and near death, the effect of the drugs on me almost fatal. I'd had my stomach pumped out, been given drugs to stabilise me, had twice been given emergency resuscitation to keep me alive. I had remained unconscious for twenty-four hours; then, when I had begun to recover consciousness, I had suffered paradoxical delirium, making no sense to anyone, rambling nonsense about not wanting to be beaten, about Nikki and Skip, both of whom I sobbed for, and ironically had to be sedated to keep me quiet until the effects of the barbiturate and Haloperidol overdose had been flushed out of my system.

Now I just lay in my bed on the children's ward, and was utterly miserable and despondent. My mother had tried to kill me. She had almost succeeded, and I owed my life to Margaret Nutt. But now I was suffering horrific flashbacks and nightmares. It seemed to me that whenever I fell asleep I had the same nightmare, despite the sedative the nurses gave me to try to minimise my disturbances.

'Am I going mad again?' I wondered. 'Am I going to end up back at Pen-y-Fal?'

These thoughts terrified me almost as much as my fear of my mother. I just did not want this life any more; it was almost more than I could bear. Perhaps it would have been better if I had not been rescued.

After a few days in hospital Sally Martin had visited me, and it was from her that I learned of how I had been miraculously saved.

On the day my mother had tried to kill me, she had indeed confronted Margaret Nutt on her doorstep, had been waiting for her upon her return from taking Peanut to school. She had ranted and raged at Margaret, and despite my opinion that Margaret was a soft sort of person, she had hidden strength. Realising my mother was mentally unstable, she had refused to discuss the matter, refused to rise to the bait when she was called a whore and accused of having an affair with my father. She had not stood arguing with my mother, who screamed and shouted in the street. She had just firmly pushed past, entered her house, and closed the door in my mother's face.

My mother, frustrated in her desire to have the matter out on Margaret Nutt's doorstep, had shouted and banged on the door for twenty minutes, before finally getting in her car and driving off with a squeal of tyres, watched by Margaret from an upstairs window.

Margaret, who had been told by my father how very unstable and dangerous his wife was, had an uneasy feeling about the situation. She had therefore telephoned Mr Beavan, the headmaster at Kings, to ask if I was at school. It had taken just ten minutes for Mr Beavan to telephone Margaret back to tell her I was not. Despite her fear that she was meddling, Margaret told Mr Beavan she was concerned for my safety. To give Mr Beavan his due, he immediately took action. He telephoned Sally Martin and told her of the situation, told her Margaret Nutt was sure I was in danger – what sort of danger he did not know – but that my mother was very unstable and quite capable of anything.

Sally Martin acted promptly. She immediately left the office and drove out to my house.

To start with my mother refused to answer the door, but Sally was not to be put off; my mother's car was in the drive so she knew my mother was at home. After a lengthy process, during which Sally called to my mother through the letterbox, my mother eventually answered the door.

Sally demanded access to me, telling my mother that Mr Beavan had telephoned her to tell her I was not at school. My mother was furtive, initially refusing to admit Sally into the house. It was only when the social worker informed my mother that she would call the police if she did not let her in, that my mother relented and allowed her in. However, she began rambling incoherent nonsense that she had returned from taking my sisters to school to find I'd taken a barbiturate overdose, and she was just about to call for an ambulance.

Sally ran to the sitting room to find me on the floor, completely unconscious, my breathing shallow and pulse irregular and faint. By now my mother was almost hysterical, insisting it was not her fault I had taken an overdose, but Sally pushed past her to get to the telephone and summon an ambulance.

The ambulance had arrived within ten minutes and I was rushed, siren blaring and with Sally Martin accompanying me, to the University Hospital of Wales.

All this had taken place ten days ago. In that time I had not seen my mother once, and with my slow recovery, not only physically but mentally too, I waited for my father to come, for I knew he'd be home soon. My only visitor had been Sally Martin, who came on the first occasion armed with a Polaroid camera to photograph my face, my black eye and bruising. Then she had obtained a letter from the hospital doctor that detailed how I had been nearly fatally overdosed.

Thereafter Sally had come every other day to see me, bringing bars of chocolate and assuring me that my mother would never be able to hurt me again. Since I'd been given these promises in the past I was somewhat sceptical. I would have to go home sometime, I knew, and that only added to my dejection, my sense of impotence in the face of someone who hated me with maniacal fervour. I could still hear my mother's screams of 'I hate you! I hate you!' echoing in my mind, and at this I'd become very distressed.

Eventually, after what seemed an eternity, one day Sally appeared on the ward with a man walking behind her. It was only when they were within a few feet of my bed that the man stepped from behind her, and I found myself gazing into my father's face.

With Sally standing at the foot of my bed, my father pulled up a chair. He gazed into my face for a long time, taking in my fading black eye, the last hints of bruising and my split lip that was yet to fully heal. When he eventually spoke, he was full of contrition; giving me promises that he would never leave me with my mother again, never leave me in danger again.

At this Sally interrupted, telling me that I would not be going home. I was going to live with my grandmother for the immediate future.

My father clutched my hand. He would never allow my mother to threaten or hurt me again, he reiterated. He looked at Sally, their eyes betraying the fact that they must have already discussed my case before coming to see me. Sally looked very determined, and I got the impression that my father was on the defensive.

'You're safe now,' he repeated. 'Mum will never, ever, hurt you again.'

How could I say that I'd heard this all before? But I looked deep into his eyes, and realised he really meant it, whatever the cost. My mother had nearly killed me this time; she had gone a step too far. She could not defend her position. She had been caught red-handed.

I nodded my assent, and my father smiled, leaning forward to hug me.

'Come on,' he said. 'You're to be discharged today, and I've brought you some clothes. It's time you went home – to your grandmother's – where you are going to live for the moment, certainly for the next few months, at least ...'

I got out of bed. The curtain was pulled to give me some privacy, while Dad and Sally stood in the ward, and I got dressed. While I pulled on my clothes, my mind was filled with thoughts of the future.

Was I going to be safe from now on? Was my mother never to be allowed near me again?

I hoped so, and by the time I pulled the curtain, dressed

and ready to leave, I was sure – certain this time – that my mother would never be able to hurt me again. Perhaps this last episode, as terrible as it had been, would finally turn out to be my salvation. I still wasn't sure, for that word – 'perhaps' – had many connotations, but I was filled with optimism as I left the ward with my father and Sally.

I had this gut instinct that as one door was closing behind me, another had just opened, one that would lead to a brighter, happier, and more optimistic future.

CHAPTER 14

A Normal Boy

The sound of the big-band era – clarinets, saxophone, trumpets, and trombones – played the introduction to the Duke Ellington song on the old 78 on my grandmother's record player, before Martha Tilton began to sing '*I let a song go out of my heart …*'

It was Christmas Day morning, 1976, and my grandmother and I were in her sitting room, awaiting the arrival of my father. We'd had bacon and eggs for breakfast, had exchanged presents, and now my grandmother had her favourite record playing.

I will always associate that music of the 1940s with my grandmother, particularly the song 'I Let a Song Go Out of My Heart', which had been my grandparents' 'special tune'. It seemed to me that the song was played over and over again that winter of 1976. As the autumnal rain became the sleet of December, still the record played on, echoing through the house as my grandmother cleaned, cooked, and knitted. She was happier than I think I had ever seen her, certainly since the death of my grandfather. I think that because I was now living with her she had a renewed purpose in life. It was as if the years dropped away from her, and beyond her white hair and wrinkles I suddenly saw what sort of a woman she had been in the 1940s: quite a looker in her mid-thirties, and full of fun.

On the November morning I left the University Hospital of Wales with my father, my grandmother was extremely gentle and kind to me. My father had finally told my grandmother the truth: how my mother had hated me and tried to kill me. Well, perhaps not the whole story; not even my father was to ever learn the *whole* story of what my mother had done to me over the years.

In the first days and weeks following my discharge my nerves failed: my stutter returned, and my nights were extremely bad again and full of nightmares. I wondered if I was falling mentally ill again, and that really frightened me. Concerned, my father had taken me to see Dr Evans at Whichurch Hospital, and the psychiatrist was able to put my and my father's minds at rest. He did not think these were signs of recurring psychosis. It was just that I had again been traumatised, and since my nerves were extremely fragile anyway, this, allied to my post-traumatic stress disorder, had weakened my mental state. Dr Evans's advice to my father was to let me relax at my grandmother's house, safe in the knowledge it was a place where I would not be hurt or endangered.

'Give him time to heal,' Dr Evans told my father. 'Bring him back to see me after Christmas.'

I continued to live with my grandmother, visited every day by my father, and I began to let my guard down, realising I was safe. I did not return to school that autumn term, but saw Peanut every weekend, was allowed to do what I wanted, when I wanted, without fear of attack or retribution.

That winter of 1976 my father had to fight hard to stop the wheels of justice moving against my mother. Sally Martin had been at the forefront of this legal assault. However, after much discussion, my father persuaded me not to make any statement against my mother, assuring me that I would from now on live with my grandmother. He also managed to obtain a doctor's letter that stated his wife was mentally unstable. Sally had wanted my mother prosecuted for assault if not attempted murder, but that would have been very difficult to prove. Without my cooperation Social Services could do nothing except serve my parents with a court order that I was never to be left alone with my mother, ever, until I reached the age of seventeen.

My father and I had some long talks that winter of 1976, as he explained his predicament to me. 'Should I divorce your mother?' he asked me, as if it was in some way my decision, which of course it absolutely was not. My father was a man with very old-fashioned morals, and in his view marriage was sacrosanct. He had loved my mother when he had married her. He was sure that beneath the surface of his mentally troubled wife of the seventies, the same uncertain and frightened woman still existed. There was no doubt by now that he could, with Sally Martin's support, gain sole custody of Vicky and Ingrid, but it was not in his heart to throw my mother out of the house, penniless and with no one to help her. Divorce was not so common in the seventies; a certain stigma still existed about it. In my father's own words, he said he had 'married *confarreatio*'. *Confarreatio* was a very ancient practice, the strictest form of marriage in the Roman world: i.e. for better or worse. This meant that whatever the circumstances, my father felt he was bound to my mother for life. He would not abandon her. Her hatred of me was, he was sure, a sign that she was mentally ill; she was a sick woman who needed help, even if sometimes that help was very difficult to give.

On Dr Evans's advice to my father that he should spend a lot of time with me, therapeutic interaction, my father decided that winter of 1976 to take me birdwatching with him every Sunday. Within a few weeks of my coming out of hospital, every Sunday the two of us began to go early in the morning out into the countryside, or along the coast to salt marshes and estuaries.

My father was very knowledgeable about birds, recognising every sort, knowing each and every call and song long before he saw them. I must admit I was never that enthralled, but my memories of the winter of 1976 and spring 1977 are of cold frosty Sunday mornings with my father, and a companionship I'd never really experienced before; a companionship that had not really existed even after we returned from West Germany.

We began to bond. Dad would talk for hour after hour on subjects as diverse as politics, art, ornithology, and history.

I had always known my father possessed a prodigious intellect, but his knowledge on all these subjects astonished me. Realising that for the first time I was more or less being treated as an equal, I found myself going to the library every week in search of books so that I could not only keep up with what he wanted to talk about, but also to contribute something to our conversations. At first my strategy was not entirely successful, for I did not know where to start, and spent hours flitting from subject to subject, desperate to consume something – anything – and remember it. Then I found my forte – history, particularly ancient history.

I began to consume everything I could find on Rome and the classical world, and I was at least able to contribute something new to the conversation. Suddenly seeing that his son was not mentally impaired as the psychiatrists had originally declared, gave my father new heart – optimism that I could and would develop. He therefore encouraged me to learn as much as I could, posing questions to me about the Roman republic – its civil wars, the Sulla dictatorship, Julius Caesar, and so on – and by the next time we talked I had the answers to his questions.

In January 1977 I returned to education at Kings, back into 3B along with Peanut, and things started to become more settled as the school-run arrangement between my father and Margaret was restored. There was no fear of my mother for me any longer, for without her interference, her insane obsessions, I knew I was safe. I had not seen her once since she'd tried to kill me in November, and she had not even sent me a Christmas card, let alone attempted any communication. This did not trouble me in the least, for without her in my life I was beginning to feel secure for the first time.

Some children find education easy, even enjoyable. I never did. It was always a struggle for me, not merely to try to catch up, but because I never seemed to have any aptitude for maths, physics, or chemistry: anything technical, in fact. Art, on the other hand, I enjoyed, and the same went for history and geography. These subjects were tangible for me, something I could see in my mind's eye.

I worked hard that spring of 1977, and as a reward for trying at school, my father agreed that I could go on holiday for a week at Easter with Peanut and Margaret. We only went to stay in a guest house in Aberystwyth in West Wales, but it was actually the first 'proper' holiday I ever had. Daily, Margaret would take Peanut and me out in her Mini to visit beaches, waterfalls, the picturesque villages, and in the late afternoons we would stroll Aberystwyth's promenade and have fish and chips while we looked out to sea. I knew that my father saw that I was getting better mentally and physically. I'd not had a petit mal since December, my stutter was fading away, and even my nights were better, although I still took the anti-psychotic, Haloperidol, and a sedative to help me sleep at night.

In June of 1977, my father took me with him to Israel, where he was acting as a discreet intermediary for the Israelis to President Sadat of Egypt. For me that trip was a defining moment of my adolescence. My previous flight had been as a sedated and damaged child from Greece to West Germany, and I hardly remember the experience. On this occasion, at Israeli government expense, we flew El Al first class, and were met at Ben Gurion Airport and driven by a chauffeur to a stunning top hotel in Tel Aviv, where my father had a suite all to himself. I now found myself living a jet-set lifestyle, so different to just two years before, when I had been locked away in an asylum and abandoned by everyone except my father. I found myself dwelling on this, and kept having to pull myself back to my new existence. I owed my father my entire life, in many more ways than one: I owed him for his perseverance to prove I could lead a normal life, and I owed him for the life I now had.

Menachem Begin had won the Israeli Premiership in the May elections of 1977. My father had up to now been working discreetly for the previous premier, Yitzhak Rabin. On our first day in Israel, my father took me with him to a substantial house north of Tel Aviv, where he met with Rabin, a man frustrated that he had not been able to secure a peace deal with Sadat before the elections. I was permitted to be present at that discussion, out on a terrace with glass of orange juice in hand. I heard Rabin state that if he'd managed to secure peace, he was sure he could have won the general election (as a postscript, Rabin became Prime Minister again in 1992, and he signed a peace deal with Yasser Arafat and the Palestinians; he was assassinated on 4 November 1995 by a radical Israeli for making peace with the Arabs).

On the following day, a chauffeured car collected my father and me and we were driven to a large villa, where I was stunned to meet Moshe Dayan, the bald man with an eye patch who was an iconic Israeli personality of the seventies. On becoming Prime Minister, Menachem Begin had made Dayan his Foreign Minister, and now my father had been summoned to tell him all about Rabin's big secret – that he'd been trying to negotiate a peace treaty with President Sadat and the Egyptians ever since 1975.

I'd been puzzled when my father had told me to pack my school uniform and bring it with me to Israel. Now all was explained when, smartly dressed, I found myself introduced to this formidable figure of Israeli politics, and was immediately taken by his genuine smile, my hand shaken, before he sat talking with my father.

As is always the case, people lead two lives. They become someone different when at work and not at home. I now saw this facet of my father for the first time. I had seen a hint of it at the Rabin meeting, but was intrigued at the different man he became, as he talked to Dayan. Dayan asked all the questions. My father gave the answers. I had only ever seen the 'home side' of my father, a man who had often been reluctant to challenge my mother, a man who had always tried to find ways to head off confrontation. Now I sat and listened to a man who was forceful and firm. At one point Dayan asked my father if Begin could go public about the secret talks, and by this means force Sadat to the negotiating table.

'No, that would be a disaster,' I remember my father

replying emphatically, slapping his hand on his thigh. 'Begin can't do that! If you do, there will never be peace, because Sadat won't be able to bring his own people on side. It has to be done discreetly. We're still a long way from going public.'

My father and Dayan talked all afternoon, and as I sat out of the way, listening to diplomatic jargon, my interest began to wane. I gazed about Dayan's living room at his large collection of antiquities, for Dayan was a keen amateur archaeologist.

At the end of their meeting, before we left, Dayan once more became the relaxed host. He'd noticed me looking at his collection, and he now showed me some of his more interesting artefacts. Finally, he came to a two-handled bowl of great antiquity.

'Do you know what this is?' he asked me.

'Yes, it's a first-century BC *krater*,' I said, giving the artefact its correct name. It was more luck than in-depth knowledge, for I had by chance seen a similar artefact in a book I'd borrowed recently from the library.

Dayan's single eye opened wide in surprise, and a broad smile played across his face. He looked at my father.

'Look after that boy, Peter,' he said. 'We've got a budding archaeologist in our midst.'

On our way back to the hotel, my father was full of pride and optimism. His meeting had gone well. Yet, I think, he was even more pleased that he had at last a son he was proud of. Many years later he told me that it was during that Israeli trip that he saw that I was capable of independence; that I would, with adulthood, become a self-sufficient individual, something that not so many years before he had been told would never happen.

I finished the summer term at Kings, and my father laid a treat on for me, as a reward for trying hard at school and as a means of expanding my interest in archaeology. He had a word with the head of archaeology at Cardiff University, Peter Webster, and made arrangements for me to participate in an archaeological excavation at Cardiff Castle that August.

Cardiff Castle is an extravagant Victorian reconstruction of an original series of castles dating back to Roman times. It is located in the city centre and is big enough to hold military tattoos in. However, beneath the neatly trimmed grass lie the remains of medieval Cardiff, and beneath that the original Roman fortress and settlement.

And so it was that during the long hot summer of 1977 I had my first taste of real archaeology, of uncovering cobbled streets, broken walls, the odd pot shard here and there. The high-point came for me when I alone was lowered down an old well, where I spent a week digging up pot shards, coins, and the fragments of glassware, for as the smallest person on the dig, only I could fit down the well, a rope secured about my waist to pull me up in case the well collapsed.

I went back to Kings in September 1977, full of stories of my adventures for my friends, happier and, at fourteen years old, more contented than I had ever been. I had become extremely close by now to Peanut and his mother, and between them, life with my grandmother and my weekends with my father, I was really enjoying life at long last. I was no star pupil at Kings, but rather was about average, I suppose, which was enough for me to keep up with everyone else.

Despite this happy life, it was decided in November 1977 that I could receive limited supervised visits from my mother. She was allowed to come to see me at my grandmother's house, but under no circumstances was I to be left alone with her. On the first visit Sally Martin insisted on being present, and told me that at the first sign of any upset by me, the first sign of distress, she would ask my mother to leave. That first meeting with my mother was very difficult for me; in fact I had to fight hard to hide my anxiety.

My parents duly came one Friday afternoon, and my anxiety mounted as I heard my mother's voice in the hall before she came into the sitting room. My main impression of that first meeting in a year was the look of astonishment on her face that I was a normal teenager. In the year since she had last seen me I had at last sprouted in growth. Although I'd never be a giant, being on the slight side, I was no longer a small and weedy child who looked several years younger than I actually was. I had lost my stutter, and I could hold a conversation with no hints at all of the mental aberrations that had been such a prevalent feature of my life since I was eight.

After a few minutes, my grandmother felt she should offer to make my mother a cup of tea. Nervously, my mother smiled and nodded. Weighing up the situation, Sally Martin used that as the excuse to go to the kitchen with my grandmother, leaving me with my parents to talk. While my father deliberately put himself in the background, my mother began to talk to me, saying she had heard I was back at school and working hard, that I had been to Israel with my father. I think I was just as nervous as she was, but I chatted to her freely, knowing I was safe. I told her about my adventures of the last year, about school, about Israel, about my dig at Cardiff Castle.

The meeting lasted just an hour that first time, and after that my father brought her to see me on Saturday afternoons once a fortnight, as we began to get used to each other. After a few months my parents began to bring Vicky and Ingrid too, and as a family we'd have tea with my grandmother. The only difference between this and a normal gathering was that I didn't go home with them; at the end of the visit I stayed at my grandmother's house.

In June 1978, just a few days after my fifteenth birthday, Sally Martin agreed that I could move back into the family home with my parents and sisters. I had visited the house a few times in the seven months since I had begun to see my mother again, but the home that I returned to live in seemed astonishingly different to the one I had left by ambulance in November 1976. There was the same wallpaper, carpets, and furniture, but it was the atmosphere that had changed. It was no longer a place of fear for me, and it was clear that my father had asserted his authority over his family. My mother was no longer the dominant force. To my eyes she seemed to have mellowed. Now that she could see – had been told – that I had no mental illness, no impairments such as autism, which had been a misdiagnosis, been given the all-clear and no longer psychotic, not even taking

Haloperidol any more, she made an effort to build a bridge to me, to be tolerant and considerate. I would never know, of course, but I think it is possible that she came to realise that her meddling with psychiatric drugs on me, her abuse of me as a young child, had caused all my problems to start with.

I let my guard down, inch by inch, and found there was little to fear. It was as if her hatred of me had been finally extinguished. However, I was still wary of her, despite her efforts at reconciliation. It was just not within me to ever forgive her for the hell she had made of my childhood. When someone tries to kill you, a barrier forms between you and that person that in no way can ever be brought down. By mutual and unspoken consent we kept a distance between us, made all the more manifest by the court order that was in place that forbade my father from ever leaving me alone with my mother in the house. This rule stayed in place until my seventeenth birthday.

I took my A levels, and by now my mother was full of pride that I was passing my exams. She seemed to want to build a 'bridge' of forgiveness to me, and for my eighteenth birthday she gave me a present of driving lessons. Yet despite these outward signs of amnesty between us, we kept our distance, and we never hugged. All these years later she would still shrink away from me, just as she had done ever since I was six years old.

When I finished school, I went to Cardiff University to study Classics and Archaeology. For most people the experience of university is an expansion of their personality; they move away from home, they make new friends, they start a new social life, and they develop beyond their parents' home. In my case, I stayed living at home, partly for practicality, partly, I have to say, because I felt my father still needed my company. I just did not have the heart to leave him alone with a woman still capable of insane rages, albeit much less frequent than they had been in the past.

To my mother's disgust, Vicky abandoned her expensive education, and left school with a handful of O levels, having no intent to pursue education or career, but far more interested in boys and partying. Perhaps it was my mother's disappointment with Vicky that finally turned her mind, her life's work frustrated and come to nothing. She began to become very odd: obsessive, secretive, and often not talking for days.

As the years rolled on, my mother's mental state was evidently in decline. She again took to using aliases, as she had done in the sixties, and began to pick insane arguments with my father.

By 1984 I was still living at home while I was at university. Ingrid was by now eleven. After a furious argument with Mother, Vicky had moved out of the house under a cloud of hate and bitter recrimination to live with her boyfriend. My mother never forgave Vicky for abandoning the ambitions for her that Vicky didn't share. In much the same way as in Stalin's Russia, we now lived in a house where Vicky became a 'non-person'. Mere mention of Vicky would induce titanic tantrums from my mother; it was a situation best avoided. Result: Vicky was never mentioned.

By now the situation in the family home had reversed. *I* was seen as the sane one, and she at long last recognised as the psychotic.

On one occasion I was alone in the house with my mother and came down the stairs to find her waiting for me in the hall, carving knife in hand. Tears streaming down her face, she began screaming at me that she wanted her children back, demanding to know who I was and why was I in her house. I beat a hasty retreat out of the front door. I fled to a telephone box to call my father at the university, telling him to come home at once because Mother had completely lost her mind. We very cautiously entered the house, prepared for literally anything, only to find my mother, composure restored and quite at ease, sitting in the kitchen reading a magazine. Deftly, my father asked her if she was okay, offered to make her a cup of tea; it was evident she had no memory of the event at all, just an hour earlier.

This incident took place in early April 1984. Concerned that my mother was losing her mind, my father secretly went to see our GP, who, to my father's surprise, expressed his gratitude that my father had finally gone to see him. With some agitation, the doctor told my father that my mother was infatuated with him, that she had been sending him presents and assertions of love for months. Utterly flabbergasted by this revelation, my father asked what should be done.

The doctor was of the opinion that my mother most likely had schizophrenia, like her brother and sister. He went further, and told my father that he was of the opinion that she should be in a psychiatric hospital, perhaps under section. Aghast, my father could not face taking that decision.

'Okay,' said the doctor. 'Come back to see me next week. We'll take a decision then.'

My father had met the doctor on Tuesday, 17 April. However, on returning home from the university on the following afternoon, my father found a note on the kitchen table from my mother that said: '*Gone. Goodbye. Voula.*'

This situation caused a lot of anxiety and distress to my father, and both he and I telephoned everyone we could think of in an effort to find her. It was all to no avail. A check of her private papers found almost everything gone, including her passport and the joint bank book that held my father's retirement fund, a sum of £20,000. An urgent visit to the bank revealed that my mother had withdrawn the entire £20,000 over the past three weeks.

On Sunday morning we were astonished when we heard the front door slam, and there stood my mother, back from wherever she had been, and dressed like a teenager, looking very strange indeed. My father kept his head, and in a level voice could only say, 'Oh, there you are. Would you like a cup of coffee?'

While my mother took her case upstairs, my father, Ingrid and I had a hurried, urgent conversation in the kitchen. Whispering, he told me and Ingrid to behave as if nothing had happened, and, once Ingrid went upstairs to see her mother, told me that he would see the doctor at the first opportunity next week to set the wheels in motion to arrange her admission to a psychiatric hospital. She had evidently lost her mind.

Those next few days were very tense. I stayed at home to keep an eye on my mother, while my father went to work. By Wednesday morning my mother had worked herself up into a frantic state, repeatedly asking me, pleading with me, to return her children. It was as if she could not reconcile herself to the fact that we'd grown up. I managed to calm her down by lunchtime, making her soup and getting her to drink it. I popped upstairs to get something, and when I returned to the kitchen I found her waiting for me with the carving knife in hand. She thrust it at me, screaming that she hated me.

At first I didn't understand what she was talking about. Then she began calling me mental, stating that she'd never wanted me, that I'd always been a distraction from my sisters for my father. With my hair prickling on the back of my neck I suddenly realised she was talking to me as if I were ten years old.

'Autistic!' she screamed at me at the top of her lungs. 'I *hate* you!'

I tried to pacify her, all to no avail.

'I never wanted you,' she screamed. 'I hate you. I hated you in Greece, and I hate you here! You should have stayed in the institution where I put you.'

Then she made the greatest mistake of her life …

'I hate you! I was kind to you, but you never gave me any gratitude, no love.'

It was at this point I snapped. I killed her. I killed her as surely as if I had plunged that carving knife deep into her heart, and it took a mere seven words.

'I remember *everything* you did to me!' was all I said.

My mother's eyes went like saucers; perhaps the first expression I had ever seen in them. She gave a scream of terror, then threw the carving knife at me, which hit me flat on the chest and fell harmlessly to the floor. She placed her hands over her ears, screaming, 'Lies! Lies! It's all lies!' She ran from the kitchen and up the stairs. I caught a fleeting glimpse of her face as she fled up the stairs. The look in her eyes was one I had never seen before, and hope to never see again.

Heart pounding, I picked up the knife and hid it in the washing machine.

Within moments my mother was back down the stairs, coat on, and handbag in hand. She pushed past me, tears streaming down her face, and all the while saying, 'Lies! Lies! Oh, it's all lies!'

But I knew *she* knew it was all true. The ECT had not eradicated my memory, and now she knew I remembered *all* the things she had done to me as a child.

She slipped past me, ran out through the front door, and was gone.

On my father's return, the news that my mother had fled again was met with some resignation. He'd been to see the doctor, who had told him that Mother would need to be seen by a psychiatrist before she could be sectioned. All that was now academic with her gone. We sat up drinking coffee all that first night, waiting for her to come back. We then began the routine of telephoning everyone we could think of; all to no avail. She had completely vanished.

Eventually, three days later, there was a knock on the door, and a policeman came to tell my father that my mother had been found. She'd taken herself by train to Folkestone. There she had booked into a hotel, and at some time during the first night committed suicide.

Driving my father to Ashford Hospital in Kent to identify my mother's body was one of the hardest things I ever had to do; his cry on seeing his wife laid out (I gave him dignity and stayed behind the curtain) the most heart-breaking sound I ever heard. My father had been through hell to rescue me from Greece, so my efforts for him that day – regardless of how hard it was for me to stay strong, so hard for me to help him back out to the car and then drive him home a widower – was the least I could do for him.

By the time of my mother's funeral a fortnight later my father had regained most of his composure, but the mourners at her funeral were pathetically few. My mother was cremated, but this presented my father with a dilemma. What shall I do with her ashes? he asked me in a whisper that night, almost as if he were afraid to ask the question out loud.

It is said that in times of crisis people can find an inner strength to be strong for others. Such an instance was now to take place for me. My father was shattered by the fact his wife had committed suicide, felt guilty that he had been unable to save her from herself. Vicky was distraught and unjustly blamed herself, for she had not visited her mother in many months. I felt guilty for having told my mother that I remembered my childhood. In our own way, we all three blamed ourselves for what happened. That was my mother's legacy to us all. All, that is, except Ingrid, who at eleven years old had never been a target, and was not yet old enough to understand that when someone dies, it's for good; they don't come back.

The night my father asked me what to do with my mother's ashes I had an inspired idea. Even in their most difficult periods my parents had talked fondly of their honeymoon in Torquay, on the south coast. My mother had a horror of graveyards, hence her desire to be cremated. So I suggested to my father that my mother's ashes be buried at sea. A telephone call the next morning to the funeral directors revealed this was not an uncommon practice, and they could even provide a lead-weighted casket specifically for the purpose.

A week after my mother's funeral, I drove my father and sisters to Torquay, where I had booked a boat to take us a few miles out to sea. In the back of my estate car reposed my mother's casket, and four wreaths.

On a bright sunny spring afternoon, three miles south of Torquay, the water beautifully clean and crystal blue, my father said a few words, then leaned out over the back of the boat and let the casket drop into the sea. There was a loud splosh, and the last we four saw of it was the silver name-plate as the casket vanished amid a cloud of bubbles down into the deep. We placed our wreaths on the water, the sailor started the engine, and we headed back to land. We four stood in silence at the back of the boat, watching as the wreaths vanished in the distance.

An episode of our lives was finally over. My mother was dead and gone. It was a very sad and final end to a life, a life that had had such a dramatic effect on me. I knew as I watched the wreaths vanish from sight that my life was now mine to make of it what I could, and it would be a life my mother could never have envisaged for me. I did not know what life would hold in store for me; no one ever does. It seemed to me that it was not only a chapter closing behind me, it was the completion of a book. A new book was about to start, and I would be the author of my own future. I was free at last.

Epilogue

It was a bright spring morning; the last gale of winter came off the Atlantic with the air full of spray and spume as I stood on the quayside at Mousehole, in the far west of Cornwall. The air was fresh against my face, my ears full of the roar of the sea. I stood alone, reflecting upon my childhood, contemplating memories I had found so hard to put down on paper.

Earlier that morning I hired a local fishing boat to take me a mile out to sea to place a wreath upon the sea for my parents; it is a mark of respect that I have maintained for twenty years, a lone yearly vigil. It turned out that the decision to bury my parents at sea was a fortuitous one, for wherever I am in the world, all I have to do is hire a boat to take me out to sea, and I can pay my respects to my long-dead parents ...

After my mother's death I stayed living at home with my father as he got older. Ingrid left to live with Vicky as soon as she was of an age to leave home, and then it was just me and my father, rattling about in that great big house. I felt like a guest at a long finished dinner party, the sort of guest who's first to arrive and the last to leave.

My father and I led a quiet life, in a subdued way, for although we had long conversations about history, art, politics, and current affairs, there were certain subjects my father would not – could not – bring himself to discuss. He would talk a lot about his life, his career, his early years with my mother, but there was a cut-off point about his relationship with my mother he would not discuss. Yet, somehow, inevitably, my father always returned to the same subject: how had my mother been able to kill herself? It was beyond his comprehension, and he never came to terms with her suicide.

With an irony that was not lost upon me, I tried to comfort him, tried to gently explain to him that she was mentally ill and so it was not possible to rationalise my mother's insane logic, her obsessions, vindictiveness, or, ultimately, her decision to kill herself.

We began to take holidays abroad, something my mother never really wanted to do, and predominantly we headed to North Africa, my father having a fascination with the climate, the culture, the birds and wildlife of a different continent. All these years later my sleep was still unsettled, and I would often wake up at two or three in the morning, go out on to my balcony for some fresh air, only to find my father out on his balcony, where he was spending the night gazing up at the star canopy. Sometimes we'd exchange a few words, more often I'd retreat to my room to give him his privacy.

On one occasion, in 1989, on holiday in the sweltering Tunisian heat of August, I got up about one o'clock in the morning and went out on to my balcony. My father heard me and came over to lean on his railing. He looked at me for a long moment, then lit a cigarette. His health was failing by now; he had lost a significant amount of weight in the last few months, and I was becoming increasingly concerned. He turned his gaze back to the Sahel, that region of fertility and palm trees north of the Sahara, as he began to talk. My father talked for the rest of the night as I stood there, telling me everything about my mother, how he had not taken a firm enough stand against her, how he should have called in a psychiatrist in the early seventies when he realised she had a form of madness he had no experience in coping with. He realised now, with hindsight, that my mental illnesses of childhood had been a manifestation of *her* illness. I had been the target; I was the one who had been made ill, almost to the point of no return. He regretted that more deeply than he could say.

He worked his way through an entire packet of cigarettes that night. He talked until the first hints of an African dawn began to break on the eastern horizon. I said not one word during the four hours he talked, for I knew I was only there to listen as he, finally, unburdened his soul. In the end, he turned away, and went back to sit on his seat to watch the dawn rise. I knew it was time to leave him alone with his thoughts, remembering a past in which he'd made mistakes, and ponder those eternal 'what if?' questions he'd never find the answer to.

On our return from Tunisia, my father was finally persuaded to go to see his doctor. It was evident to me that he was very sick, and he was diagnosed with advanced chronic myeloid leukaemia. It was incurable, and he had not long left to live. Although it was a clinical illness that killed him, I think deep down my father died of a broken heart. His life had started full of so much promise, a life that had so many possibilities, only to end in disaster. It was a life in which he married a woman who, although he loved her, had turned out to be a dangerous psychopath; his son had been nearly destroyed and killed. A wife who bought his house to the brink of destruction. Then, when she realised the game was up, she took him for every penny and killed herself before she could be forced to answer in any way for her misdeeds.

After his diagnosis of leukaemia, my father insisted on sitting up all night that autumn, talking to me about his life, about my mother in the fifties and sixties, about his work in Germany, about the Middle East. It was as if my father was afraid of the nights, only content to retire to bed for a few hours once the sun had begun to rise; a small victory for him to have made each new day as it came.

My father died a very hard death a few days before Christmas 1989, and as I sat holding his hand all through his traumatic last night in the University Hospital of Wales, I found my mind going back all those years to the night I had sat holding Nikki.

Most of the people from my childhood are dead now: my mother, my father, my grandmother, Margaret Nutt, Nikki, Dr Nordbusch, Dr Schultz, and Auntie Elle. Even Uncle

Manolis is dead. He vanished overboard one winter's night the same year I was rescued from the Attica and returned to Britain. Was he in fear of what he'd done to me, in fear of retribution; had he committed suicide? Perhaps it was an accident. No one will ever know.

The only people of my childhood I'm still in touch with are Peanut and my sisters. Peanut now lives in the United States, where he's an expert on agriculture. My sisters still live in Wales, and I see them once a year for a few hours, but the collective memories of our childhood make it too uncomfortable – painful – for us to be together. They have happy lives now with husbands and children, new lives in which it is better to block out the past.

I too have a happy new life, one which my parents could never have envisaged for me. A year after my father's death I met and fell in love with Rosemary – Rosy – whom I soon married. The love Rosy and I have for each other is absolute, a true partnership; we are the best of friends. In the end it was Rosy who pushed me to my full potential. I had spent several years working as an insurance administrator, but she persuaded me that I should pursue my dream of becoming an author. In the early 1990s I took the plunge to quit my job and start a new career as a writer. It took me five years to learn how to write a book – the minutiae and skills of language usage necessary to publish – and since 1998 I have been a successful author. Deep down I have this eternal hope that my father would have been proud of my life and career; so very different from the tensions, fear, and mental illnesses of my childhood.

Despite all I've been through, I am now happily married and in a career I enjoy.

I contemplated all these things as I stood watching the raging Atlantic off the quay at Mousehole, the winds of early spring tugging at my coat and trousers. Usually I do not delve too deeply into these memories. It is something I have learnt I have to turn off to keep sane; to put a mental firewall up between me and my memories for self-protection. However, to write this book I had just spent a year delving into the sources of my nightmares. The names, places, and painful memories I have avoided thinking about ever since my childhood. In a way I think it had been a cathartic process, for me the laying to rest of many ghosts.

Somewhere far far away, I could hear a voice calling me – 'Alex … Alex … Alex …' – just as my father had done to pull me back to reality the day he rescued me from the Attica. My toes hung over the edge of the quayside, out into open space as I gazed down into the emerald-green sea as it plunged up and down, up and down; so clean, so inviting. I could see why my father had left instructions that he wanted to spend eternity with my mother buried at sea off Torquay.

My reverie – my mind lost in time – came back to the present, and I cautiously backed away from the edge. I turned and saw Rosy standing thirty yards away. She looked relieved to see me safely back from my private yearly vigil. I smiled at her, and walked back along the cob, the wind a strong hand in the small of my back propelling me along.

'Are you okay?' Rosy asked, her face anxious, hair blown, tugged and flailing around her face.

I nodded.

I took her hand and we walked into the small town. It was time to find a local pub for a coffee or something stronger.

It was time I moved on. I would never forget my past, or the people who had shaped it for good or bad. But it was, I realised, time to look ahead to the future.